THE SIRTFOOD DIET

New Step By Step Guide To Activate Your Skinny Gene, Lose Weight In A Simple Way, Burn Fat And Have A Healthier Lifestyle

ANNE-MARIE GREEN

TABLE OF CONTENTS

CHAPTER ONE

AN OVERVIEW

Weight loss and the quest for keeping a perfect body shape are universal aspirations among people around the world. With the need to burn off fat continually rising by the day, no one wants to miss out in the bid to shape down their weight, look trimmed and attractive. However, apart from the general need to wane off excess fat and cholesterol content, there are different reasons for which people crave to lose weight. Amanda's situation exemplifies one of the much more profound and far-reaching differing reasons.

Amanda, 50, is an experienced and versatile interior decorator and events planner who runs a successful business in the heart of Chicago. With a brilliant and rich engineer husband and three lovely children, her life is almost perfect! One of her kids is through with College, while the other two are doing pretty well in their respective colleges. She and her dear husband, John, live in their own house in Illinois, the mortgage fully paid for. They even manage to go on exotic vacations to Europe and the Caribbean once or twice a year.

However, Amanda doesn't seem to have it all with her health as she has an unhealthy addiction to sugary foods, just as is often the case with many Americans and individuals living in first-world countries. This is a lifestyle she had developed while she was still at College and into the early days of her career as a public accountant. Being a public accountant was quite a demanding and time-consuming role. And as a result, Amanda was always stressed because of the constant pressures that she had to deal with. Her kitchen life and routines had no space in the diary. Snacks, pastries, candy, and chocolate bars were the regular meals that she fed on to stave off boredom and help feel full at work. Kicking this habit became almost an impossible thing to do. At first, it didn't seem much like a problem, and so, it was understandable why she was not bothered by the extra pounds that she had added on within a short time.

Only a few days to her fortieth birthday, however, the reality of what she was in began to dawn on her. She had gone to have a photo studio session for her birthday when it hit her how much weight she had put on. Shocked and exacerbated by the sight of her unattractive self in the photoshoots, Amanda felt guilty for her new looks. Something had to be done to mend it up. The birthday photos served as a liberating sign for her to do something about her weight without any ado. She discussed with her doctor, who referred her to a nutritionist's place where she was advised to begin a dieting regimen that would help her cut back on her calorie consumption. The nutritionist wasn't, however, considering one fundamental problem – Amanda's debilitating addiction to sugary foods. Her new patient barely survived three weeks on the new diet when she began to sneak in chocolate cake in her bag as she went to work. Soon, she slipped off the wagon entirely and went back to her old, unhealthy eating habits.

All through her forties, Amanda had tried out several weight loss programs and popular 'magic' products. As expected, all of that soon turned out to be a waste of time, effort, and money. It wasn't the case that those regimens and products were entirely useless; the problem was that Amanda wasn't ready for them. Her situation wasn't different from that of someone who craved change but was not prepared one bit to change. She felt those health routines were forced on her so that she could suddenly and drastically cut down her calorie consumption. Now, a few months after her fiftieth birthday, her doctor has told her that she suffers a great risk of developing high blood pressure because the amount of fat in her body is beginning to take a toll on her heart, which now requires much force to pump blood around her body.

Today, there are many more Amandas in the world with even more severe conditions to cope with and deal with. At one point or the other in our lives, we consciously or subconsciously pick up the habit of over-eating foods that are rich in processed sugars but which are sadly low in essential nutrients. This habit very fast to become an addiction. It is not that we don't know what it means to be addicts. We do, but just enjoy and can't call it a quit with that which we enjoy. And because almost everyone around us seems to be doing it, we don't really care. Eventually, we get a wake-up call, while some of us do not. Either way, we tend to end up overweight, or with some health challenges as a result of our terrible over-consumption of unhealthy junk food.

This book sets out to help you build a sustainable system that will enable you to lose weight without ever feeling frustrated and falling off the wagon. At least half of overweight persons in the United States have tried some type of weight-loss regiment at one point or the other in their lives. And in most cases, these people are not able to sustain strict diets because of their addiction to binge-eating and the feeling of being full. The goal of the Sirtfood system, therefore, is to help you, through a step-by-step and day-by-day manner, to formulate a specialized diet that allows you to eat enough food to power through your daily activities while helping you to reduce body fat gradually. Simultaneously too, your body's muscle mass is maintained and duly consolidated. You can rest assured that this new formula basically allows you to lose weight without feeling starved or lethargic utterly. This unique, systematic diet is called the Sirtfood Diet.

Before moving on to describe how the sirtfood diet works, I believe it is essential at this point to review the psychology behind building a system that works instead of rushing blindly to achieve giant, lofty, and most times, unattainable goals. In dieting, and life generally, we all tend to revel in setting lots of huge vital goals for ourselves, and perhaps, for our loved ones. A student in the College may say to himself: "This semester, I want to have at least a 3.5 GPA out of the maximum possible 4.0. A car salesman may say to himself: "This month, I want to sell enough cars to make at least ten thousand dollars in commissions." A person trying to lose weight may say: "This week, I'll exercise hard, rest well and watch every single thing I eat so that by the end of the week, I would have lost at least 10 pounds." These are all relatively reasonable goals that the average individual can attain if they put in ample hard work. The complication, however, usually arises from the fact that most people are so fixated on these goals that they do not focus enough on how the day-to-day execution of their plans to achieve them would go. As a result of this misplaced priority, they end up, more often than not, failing to meet their desired targets.

Don't get me wrong; having the goal to lose ten pounds a week is a fantastic idea, and if you watch your diet and exercise quite vigorously while sleeping well too, you can actually achieve that goal. However, the only way you are going to crush that goal is if you can draft out a plan that you can follow systemically to help you achieve it. This goal is most definitely not going to complete itself. However, when you have a system in place to help you follow through your long-term academic, income, or weight goals, then your job becomes significantly more comfortable. Instead of being fixated on the ultimate final result, you become addicted to meeting your small, daily targets. And we all know that crushing small daily goals is more natural than blindly trying to chase lofty ones without a single plan in place.

The sirtfood diet is a system, not a goal. It is meant to help you develop a sustainable eating routine that doesn't motivate you to go hungry. With the sirtfood diet, you do not have to cope with constant fatigue, lethargy, lack of motivation, and eventual relapse into unhealthy eating that often comes with most diets. This is because the diet has been well-researched and adequately tested, and has been designed to help you crush your weight-loss goals comfortably, one day at a time.

When you get on with the sirtfood diet, you will practically become so obsessed with making sure that you are following the system (getting healthy can be addictive too!) that you wouldn't want to think of quitting. You'd just gaze at the mirror one day and realize how paying so much attention to following your system has helped you to attain your goals without you being so fixated on them. The process is far from being one of those one-off programs whose results only last a while.

You may wonder if the sirtfood diet is only valid for a specific set of individuals. That, of course, is usually the case with so many of the so-called diet foods around, but it is certainly not the case with Sirtfood Diet. The sirtfood diet has been proven to be effective in promoting weight loss, increased energy levels, and improved mental health among a wide variety of people. Generally, every single aspect of the population can benefit from the sirtfood diet model. Some of the most important beneficiaries of the diet, however, include:

Overweight people: If you want to determine obesity, weight is generally calculated in terms of an individual's body mass index, which is obtained by dividing the person's body mass by their weight in squared meters. Typically, adults with a BMI above $25kg/m^2$ are considered to be overweight. In comparison, individuals with a BMI above $30kg/m^2$ are considered obese and need to get to work right away on their weight lest they suffer dangerous health consequences. Generally, children and adolescents with BMIs exceeding $20kg/m^2$ need to seek adequate medical attention and advice on how to curb their weight gain and prevent far-reaching complications.

Since the sirtfood diet is designed to help people lose weight without putting too much pressure on them psychologically, physically, and financially, it is a perfect weight-loss option for slightly overweight and morbidly obese individuals. The diet is simple, contains foods that are delicious and enjoyable, and does not require an individual to go unnecessarily hungry. The availability of energy for the dieting individual and the feeling of satiation after the meals in the diet will help ensure that an overweight individual does not fall into their old, unhealthy eating habits. The exclusive collection of foods that make up the sirtfood diet and their active ingredients will then help to set off a series of reactions within the body, which will instigate rapid and sustainable weight loss. Based on all of these, the sirtfood diet can, therefore, be a reliable means to help mitigate life-threatening obesity and slightly excess weight without putting the individual under undue pressure.

Older people: Older members of the population are quite predisposed to gaining unhealthy weight, which they may find quite challenging to shed. Our mature ladies and men generally tend to engage in less strenuous or physically-demanding activities. It is the same experience for everyone in that phase of life. Hence, most of the fats they consume end up being stored within their bodies. The sirtfood diet, however, can be an enjoyable and sustainable technique to help these aged people lose weight without putting them through the undue and unrealistic rigors of extreme exercise or crippling diets. With the sirtfood diet, senior citizens can eat a selected collection of healthy foods at regular intervals to help them stay satiated and energized while losing weight and building necessary muscle mass.

Thin or Anorexic People: Understandably, you might not have thought that skinny people would be a target of a weight-loss diet, but the sirtfood diet is truly unique, and it does have something to offer everyone. The specialized chemicals that are released from the carefully selected foods that make up the sirtfood diet do not only help to burn unwanted fat; they also help to build muscle mass within the body. How on earth can the same diet plan help to reduce fat while at the same time helping to boost muscle mass? Just hold your breath and stay glued. You'll find out exactly how the sirtfood diet carries out these two seemingly contradictory functions in perfect harmony in the next couple of pages.

Fitness Enthusiasts: If you are neither overweight nor skinny but would like to get in shape and look fitter, trimmer, and more attractive, then the sirtfood diet can work wonderfully well with a light exercise regimen to help give you the body of your dreams. The sirtfood food is reputed for its ability to help decimate fat stores in the body while helping to burgeon the body's muscle mass rapidly. In any case, if you've been on the hunt, searching for the perfect set of foods that would help complement your efforts in the gym, then you have just found that very solution. Experts even have it that with the sirtfood diet, you do not necessarily have to undergo hours of rigorous exercise at the gym to gain that body shape that you have always dreamed of. With a carefully reviewed home workout schedule and running in the morning about thrice a week, you should be able to get that desired body shape carved out while, of course, integrating the sirtfood diet into your food timetable.

Young people: This is another section of the population that can benefit immensely from the merits that the sirtfood diet has to offer. Young people are usually highly-active individuals who lead pretty high-powered lifestyles. From ceaseless college lectures, through a demanding job, partying with friends, playing games and sports, and a list of such endless things are a range of activities that take up the time and energies of young people. Because of their demanding lifestyle, young people need as much energy as they can. Piling up fat in the body will naturally make an individual feel fatigued faster. The sirtfood diet can help young people, irrespective of their body size to build muscle mass, increase their energy levels daily, and help them improve their mental alertness to perform superbly well at intellectual tasks.

Career professionals: The Sirtfood Diet is another perfect fit for career professionals. If you work at a demanding segment of the economy – for instance in a hospital, a financial services firm, or you run your own small business, then you will agree with me that you can never have too much energy or alertness. Most individuals are active and alert at work in the first half of the day. Later in the day, usually from mid-afternoon, most professionals experience a drop in their energy levels, leading to a significant dip in performance and results. The sirtfood diet contains specialized natural chemical substances that will help your body to extract the maximum amount of energy possible from the natural foods you eat. It becomes interesting if all you want is to stay optimally motivated and energized throughout your day. The foods in the sirtfood diet will also help you to build muscle mass and lose weight as a busy professional, thereby helping you to be more confident and motivated at work.

Who you are don't matter, but what you do or what your performance goals are. As long as all that you want is to have more energy to help you through your daily life, or even to feel healthier and more mentally alert generally; then the sirtfood diet is the answer. It can bc a highly valuable tool to help you achieve your body goals simultaneously as you begin a journey to high performance and desired health.

Hence, as you plan to begin this journey to this new revolutionary dietary lifestyle, I'm here to make you a promise. How incredibly will it sound to you if you are told that within a week of sticking religiously to this sirtfood diet, you will lose at least 5 to 7 pounds? That's breathtaking, isn't it? That is what you stand to experience. Within that first week, you will feel your energy levels rise noticeably, feel your moods improve, and you will experience a new, noticeable feeling of increased general wellbeing.

If you stick to this program till the end of the first month and combine it with a healthy lifestyle, such as regular moderate exercise and a healthy lifestyle, you would sooner than expected feel nauseated by the urge to continue with hold addiction to unhealthy foods. Your weight loss will continue; you'll drop another few pounds of fat and increase your body's muscle mass. You will experience a profound increase in clarity and alertness at work and home, while at ditto time, your moods will improve, and so will your sleep. You will feel like you've just secured a new lease on life.

The sirtfoods immense impact on our lives is nonnegotiable because of the far-reaching effects that the foods that we put in our bodies have on our general wellbeing. Most people do not understand just how gruesome unhealthy eating habits can be on their general wellness. When you overeat sugar, saturated fats, and other unhealthy food, you pile your body with unnecessary stores of fats. These fat stores are not adequately metabolized in time because you keep eating these unhealthy foods at regular intervals. The fat stores make you feel sluggish and slow; they make it difficult to exercise and work efficiently. They may have long-term adverse effects on your health – especially on the efficiency of your cardiovascular system. When you take up a new healthy diet, you give your body fresher, cleaner fuel to run on. You can think of sirtfoods as pure energy for your body's ecosystem. The former foods you were consuming were causing pollution and only clogging up your body's landscape with unhealthy fats and harmful unwanted compounds. Once you choose to run your body on clean energy, you effectively cut off the source of the pollution. Gradually, your body will begin to let go of the toxic deposits, and your entire body system will feel rejuvenated.

The sirtfood diet, unlike most of the other specialized diets out there, is very affordable too. I've seen diet plans that force you to eke out thousands of dollars for a month's food budget. It is even more annoying to find out that these foods are complicated to prepare, or that they aren't things you can wake up in the morning, put together, and eat before going to work. Practicality and affordability are significant deciding factors in the eventual success or failure of any particular diet. All the foods that make up the sirtfood diet can be prepared from the regular food products you can purchase from your regional grocery. The recipes are also simple and straightforward, and in a matter of minutes, your food is done, you can eat and get yourself off to work or school.

The practicability of the sirtfood diet is not only in its affordability and ease of preparation; however, it's also in its ability to keep you satiated and motivated to work. The basis of most diets is to get you to consume as little food as possible. This technique helps to burn fat in the short term, but with another potential damage as it also withers the body's muscle mass and makes the individual feel lazy, less energized, and generally fatigued. The sirtfood diet basically capitalizes on you eating enough food to work, so it helps you to stay focused and helps to ward off all your unhealthy cravings effectively.

Why exactly is so much information being let out about the Sirtfood diet? You may be curious. For sure, I can confidently make massive statements about the sirtfood diet because it is a dieting regimen that has been tested to be effective and trusted to deliver results over the years. The menu itself has been designed only to include a selected variety of foods that possess exceptional properties, which lead to weight loss, muscle gain, and mental clarity. In thousands of people who have stayed committed to this tested and trusted diet system, the sirtfood diet has helped to recondition body metabolism and improve the overall quality of life.

How rapidly soon will the results of the sirtfood diet show? According to average results from a variety of studies, as mentioned earlier, you should be able to knock about 5 to 7 pounds of pure fat off your body within the first week of taking up the sirtfood diet. Within a month, you could be looking at up to 20 pounds of fat lost, and a respectable gain in muscle. Since the sirtfood diet helps to burn fat and maintain or gain muscle mass, your weighing scale may not be such an excellent tool to help judge your progress. Instead, you should watch out for signs of fat loss around your abdomen and waistline. If you find that you have to move your belt buckle up a notch, or your skirts fit better around your waist, then you may have your signs that the sirtfood diet is indeed helping you to burn fat. You will also find your ability to concentrate soar within the first few weeks of starting this diet. You will feel your home workouts translating to more muscle gain since you are now eating to synergize with your exercise, not to antagonize it. Within a month of the sirtfood diet, your sugar cravings will drop extensively, while the gradual drop in fat will have positive effects on your blood pressure.

In a pilot study conducted among 40 participants at a fitness clinic in London, England, the powers of the sirtfood diet were revealed, and they were magnificently breathtaking. It is one thing to predict the potency of these foods, and it is yet another to experience their effects within a short time frame. During the pilot study, the 20 main foods that make up the sirtfood diet were carefully combined to create the sirtfood diet for the participants. The study was carried out under strictly controlled conditions. The fitness clinic had its own in-house restaurant, so there was no need for the food to be sourced externally. A lot of the participants were already previously healthy people, so the diet had to be super-effective for it to have produced such remarkable results on them.

For seven days, the progress of these individuals who undertook the experiment was closely monitored. Their weight, changes in body composition, fat and muscle levels, and their blood sugar levels were all carefully tracked. For the first three-to-four days of the week that the study was carried out, the individuals all consumed a maximum of 1000 calories per day. This calorie restriction is necessary for the first phase of the Sirtfood diet. However, since this strict restriction only applies to the early three days of the first phase, it was quite easy for the participants to adhere to it. In the last four days of the study, the participants were allowed to consume up to 1500 calories per day. After the initial stages, you can up your calorie consumption as long as you are not consuming prohibited foods.

Of the 40 individuals who began the sirtfood diet, 39 were able to complete it, representing a 97.5% adherence rate. Unarguably, there is a 97.5% chance that you would be able to at least make it through the first phase of this incredible diet. And if you make it through the first week, which is the most challenging part, transitioning to the more natural second phase where you get to eat even more would not be such an arduous task. When the fat and muscle statistics of the 39 people who completed the study were checked, the result showed that the group lost an average of 7 pounds of fat in the first week. Most of them maintained their muscle mass, or even gained a bit more. This muscle gains and feeling of satiety is what makes the sirtfood regimen so outstanding and unique. On average, each participant was found to have lost reasonable fat around the waistline and abdominal region. The average participant didn't complain of hunger since the diet has been designed to keep you satiated and energized while burning fat. The average participant reported greater vigor and drive to work and attack their daily goals. What's more, within a week, most of these excited participants were already looking quite trimmer than they did at the start of the regimen.

So, what particularly do you hope to gain from this sirtfood diet? In the nearest future, if you stick to the sirtfood diet regimen as religiously as possible, this diet will help you achieve a couple of exciting life goals. Imagine a future where you don't have to worry about your unhealthy sugar cravings again because you are energized continuously and satiated by your consumption of healthy food. Think of a future where you are just randomly walking in the park, and someone who knew you from a year ago walks up to you and can't believe their eyes because all your fat has been transformed into stable, healthy muscle.

Picture that future where every time you visit the doctor, you get a clean bill of health instead of a warning that your heart might buckle under the strain of your fat soon. Visualize the future where you head to work filled with a power meal, and you're ready to crush all your goals for the day without breaking a sweat. Imagine a future filled with fewer hospital visits, more incredible times spent with family, and better achievements at work. Think of that good time to come with a happier, healthier, and a more accomplished you. This future is what the sirtfood diet combined with a healthy lifestyle, can give you.

Now that you have a firm perception of what this book is about and the kind of life you are about to be introduced to, it is time to step things up a notch explore fully, the nitty-gritty of what precisely the sirtfood diet is about.

CHAPTER TWO

THE NITTY-GRITTY OF THE SIRTFOOD DIET

The term 'sirtfood' refers to a natural or slightly processed food item, one that contains a set of select chemicals known as polyphenols. The polyphenols in the sirtfoods can help you activate a set of genes in the body known as 'sirtuins.' These sirtuins are also known as skinny genes, and when they are activated, they can trigger weight loss in a person. That's how sirtfoods work, in a nutshell. Now, let's go a little bit into the technical details.

Most dietary plans work based on reducing the number of calories that a person consumes. This technique mostly works in theory, but it is almost always doomed to fail in the real world. Human beings are not machines or computers, and making massive, sudden changes to something as fundamental to our lives as our diet within an unimaginable short time is almost always impossible and quite hazardous if ever achieved. Most diets programs require you to rapidly cut down on the number of calories you consume per day. A lot of fitness fads are usually seen calculating the number of calories of food they think they might have ingested within a day. When followed correctly, calorie-restricting diets can make people lose weight, but that's about where the benefits stop. It just doesn't extend beyond that. A calorie-restricted diet tightly regulates the amount of food that passes into your body system. This means that your body is forced to burn its fat deposits to gain energy. Still, once those deposits are gone, then your muscle mass begins to wither slowly, instead of looking trim and fit. At the same time, on these calorie-restricting diets, a lot of people end up looking pitifully thin as their muscle mass continues to shrink and wither away. The drastic drop in calories consumed also has other immediate effects as the recipient (call them victims, if you like) constantly feels hungry, irritated, and fatigued. The phrase: "A hungry man is an angry man" comes into play quite well here.

When on a calorie-restricting diet, the entire body is placed on a limited supply of the fuel it needs to run, and yet the individual is expected to function efficiently. Doesn't that sound like a counterproductive or self-antagonism approach? The hunger and irritation that the person feels would soon begin to affect all the other aspects of their life. They may find it difficult to concentrate at work due to his new strict diet that forces him to keep close tabs on the number of calories of food they consume per day. Performing even the easiest physical tasks may become difficult, as the body slowly begins to break down. It should not come as a surprise to hear of people on these strict diets simply swooning when under intense stress and pressure since they are trying to overwork a body system that is running on fumes.

Calorie-restricting diets uncontrollably stretch their tentacles into the immune system and may predispose the individual to diseases. The foods that we eat contain essential nutrients and vitamins that help us to keep our bodies in optimal shape. Carbohydrates provide energy, and so do fats. Fat deposits can help to provide warmth. Proteins help to build muscle mass and ensure the proper replication of cells within the body. Vitamins and mineral salts serve essential functions in preventing diseases and keeping critical body organs such as the kidneys and liver in perfect shape. When people suddenly restrict their calories without giving their body system a chance to adjust gradually, the immune system can take a severe hit. The body isn't being supplied with the natural biochemical that it needs to function optimally anymore, so, it becomes vulnerable to disease from any direction.

Finally, more often than not, the strain from a calorie-restricting diet becomes too much for anyone to bear. If the person used to be addicted to sugary and junk foods before, the stress becomes even more significant to deal with. Half the time, these victims are hungry, and the only thing they can think of is dashing to the snack shop down the street and grabbing some doughnuts and a soda. Eventually, the body is just not able to take the strain anymore, and the person goes right back to their former unhealthy diet. Like a hailstorm, the fats come rushing back, and in a matter of weeks, these individuals are back right where they started – fat, unhealthy, and unhappy. It's a brutally vicious cycle – one that only a genuinely sustainable diet like the sirtfood diet can break.

Just as has been mentioned earlier, the sirtfood routine contains a variety of selected foods, mostly green leafy vegetables, whole grains, cocoa, coffee, and even dark chocolate and red wine! Unlike most of these tough unrealistic diets out there, the sirtfood routine is out to prove to the world that people can become healthier and fitter while still eating green and tasty foods. Of course, if you are going to be successful with the sirtfood diet, you are going to have to cut back on a couple of harmful foods. Still, you would be too busy enjoying the delicious new options on your new menu that you wouldn't care about the former foods that only used to stuff you up with pounds upon pounds of fat anyway.

All foods certified as sirtfood have all been extensively analyzed to help you understand their compositions and their effects on the body. One thing that has been found in all sirtfoods is that they contain a couple of compounds known collectively as polyphenols. The first sirtfood was analyzed in the 20th century and found to be the skin of red grapes that are used in making red wine. During the analysis of these skins, it was discovered that these skins contained a polyphenol known as resveratrol. It had been noted earlier that unlike people who are heavy drinkers of alcoholic drinks, people who drink red wine do not tend to get unhealthy or overweight. Instead, red wine drinkers seemed to be svelte, fit, and naturally energetic.

Scientists dug further into how resveratrol, one of the most active compounds in red wine, could be affecting the burning of fat deposits and the maintenance of a trim body figure with a moderate muscle mass within the body. Their findings were nothing short of being revolutionary. In their studies, these scientists found out that there are a set of genes located in our bodies known as sirtuins. There are seven sirtuins in total, and they all work together in a systematic way. Each of them is named in a simple manner. The first sirtuin gene is called SIRT 1, the second; SIRT 2, and the numbering goes on like that, reaching SIRT 7. SIRT 1 and SIRT 3 have been found out to be the most active genes in the family of the sirtuins.

Sirtuins are a group of genes known as inducible genes. There are several other genes located throughout the body that work using a similar mechanism as the sirtuins. They stay, relatively hidden and unnoticed within the body. However, when a condition arises that necessitates them to swing into action, inducible genes become activated. They do not just become activated magically. They are actually activated in response to the situation that necessities their attention. You can think of them like firefighters. Firemen do not just drive their trucks and come to your house. Your house has to be on fire, and you need to call their attention to the fire. The signal that's sent to the firemen in the form of your phone call then forces the fire extinguishers to spring into action to come and put out the fire – the incident that led to them getting invited in the first place. This analogy works very well with the sirtuins. Sirtuins, as a unique set of genes, remain dormant over the lives of most people because they are not activated. However, when they are activated with the right signals, sirtuins perform an extremely overwhelming function – they put the entire body in survival mode and aim to save the body, just like firefighters saving a house do. To help the body have as much energy as possible to survive the 'perilous' times that the sirtuins believe the body is in; usually, these genes burn up stores of fat within the body system to provide energy. They deploy mechanisms to repair and rejuvenate damaged cells, and they boost the abilities of the body's immune system, making the body even more resistant to disease.

Now, the big question: Why on earth would sirtuins think the body is in danger and get activated? The answer is sirtfoods. Sirtfoods contain polyphenols, and the way the regimen is designed, in your first few days of consuming sirtfoods, your calorie intake is reasonably restricted. In the early three days, your calorie intake is limited to 1000 calories, and in the last four days of the first phase, your calorie intake is kept at 1500 calories. The combination of polyphenolsinflux into the body and the drastic reduction in the consumption of calories in the first week leads to the activation of a stress pathway within the body system. This stress pathway ends in the activation of the previously dormant sirtuins genes. This is where the magic happens. Once the sirtuin genes are activated, the genes serve as directors – much like the corporate executives of a Fortune 500 company. They direct the body mechanisms under their command to burn up the stores of fat within the body to ensure that the body is supplied with the energy it needs to keep running in the wake of the restriction of calories entering the body. The sirtuins also send forth a series of signals which enable another set of mechanisms to clean out toxic materials from cells and rejuvenate ailing body cells. The sirtuins deploy another set of mechanisms to boost the body's immune system in order for the latter to protect the body against any possible attack.

Sirtuins carry out their job efficiently, as has been proven by scientific studies, and as long as the polyphenols continue to stream continuously into the body. The sirtuin genes remain activated and maintain their essential duties of directing the burning up of fats and building body cells. This action accounts for how the body gains more muscles during the placement period. As the presence of the sirtuins in your body becomes stable, the sirtuin's diet allows you to ease up on the restriction of calories gradually and to eat more food. The sirtuins have already been activated and established. Once the body is no longer under the stress of calorie restriction, and the polyphenols keep flowing in, the sirtuins bloom and become stable, steadily directing all essential functions leading to weight loss, abundant energy, muscle gain, and supercharged immunity.

For the first few days of the sirtfood diet, you can experience a couple of downsides. These downsides are especially more noticeable in the first three days of the first phase (i.e., first week) of the diet. Because of the drastic reduction of your calorie consumption to a thousand calories per day, you may experience hunger, slight irritability, and mild fatigue. These effects are only noticeably pronounced if you used to be a heavy eater. However, bear it in mind that the first three days represent the small sacrifice that you have to make for the greater good that is to come. As soon as you hit day 4, you are free to increase your daily consumption to 1500 calories, and after the first week, you can comfortably go back to eating three healthy meals per day while still keeping your sirtuins genes at work; transforming your body.

What are the foods that make up the sirtfood diet? There are quite a number of them. Twenty primary foods have been discovered to contain the concentration of polyphenols, which the body needs to activate the sirtuin genes. When these sirtfoods are combined in harmony over a period of time – their effects help to produce magical results. There are, of course, other permitted foods that also contain reasonable amounts of polyphenols, and those would be discussed in later chapters. Cocoa, extra virgin olive oil, red onions, garlic, parsley, chilies, kale, strawberries, walnuts, capers, tofu, and green tea, are some of the foods that are recommended as part of the sirtfood diet. A full list of the 20 foods that make up the sirtfood diet and their active polyphenols would be given in the adjoining pages. These foods have incredible fat burning effects and with the capacity to contribute an ample amount of essential ingredients that can also help to improve the functioning of the body system. When consumed together, these foods have a collectively spectacular effect.

You may wonder if there are evidential stats of people who have benefitted greatly from the sirtfood diet? Yes, there are. The number is not only emphatic; it is breathtaking. First, apart from a 40-man study conducted in London, several people have tried out the sirtfood diet, and have confirmed it to be a genuinely revolutionary technique to lose weight while retaining muscle and staying energized.

Adele, the famous English singer, and multiple Grammy award winner, is one of the few celebrities who swear by the power of the sirtfood diet. In the early months of 2020, Adele's social media posts have shown her to have cut down on her body fat, while she now boasts of an even trimmer and visibly more energetic look. While she was questioned about her new look and the renewed palpable zest she attacked life with, Adele had a simple answer to give: "The sirtfood diet."

Another individual who has benefitted immensely from the efficacy of the sirtfood diet is a TV sports presenter named Laura. Laura is an attractive 29-years old personality with a blossoming career. Whether we care to admit it or not, the success of the career of a person who faces millions of people daily depends quite heavily on their looks. Laura has always been a hardworking and talented TV presenter, but her stunning looks sure did add to her appeal as a TV personality. However, as Laura hit her late 20s, she noticed a strange and rather unwelcome development. She was beginning to put on some considerable weight. At first, she didn't think much about it, as it only made her curvier and rounded, but as she grew older, the weight only piled up more till she realized that she needed to do something. She confessed that she had battled a debilitating sugar addiction since her late teens. Like a lot of Americans, Laura had subconsciously integrated the habit of eating a lot of sugary snacks into her daily routine. Her work in the media industry was pretty demanding, so in between TV programs and getting ready to host a show, she found herself eating a lot of sugary snacks to stay satiated and feel energized.

It was on a matter of time as shortly afterward, her

addiction had started coming back to haunt her. She couldn't afford to lose her looks at this point in her career. Of course, she needed to look prim and fit, but she didn't just want to. One part, she enjoyed her sugary snacks pretty much to let go of them. In one of our encounters, Laura confessed to being so hooked on sugar that she carried a bottle of syrup in her handbag to apply to coffee and pastries that she felt were just not sweet enough for her liking. Did she know that excessive sugar consumption was harmful to her health? Yes. Did she care? Yes, she did. Could she willingly quit her excessive sugar consumption? Sadly, the answer to that was No.

In an attempt to proffer an effective solution to her weight problems, Laura ventured into the world of dieting. At first, she tried some of the numerous calorie-restricting diet options recommended by most weight-loss experts online and offline. In the meantime, she had managed to stay dedicated to some of these diets for a while until she just couldn't bear the strict nature of some of them. Eventually, every single time, she found herself going back to her favorite junk food, and her shape wouldn't get any better. Laura felt helpless, but then, her search and frustration soon stopped as she discovered the sirtfood regimen.

Within two weeks of eating sirtfoods, Laura's cravings had dipped. This was the first breakthrough for her. To prevent her from gaining even more weight, she always felt guilty of consuming too many calories, but just couldn't help the junk snacks. However, with the sirtfood diet, she was free to eat enough food to get her satiated –which wasn't a lot. This translated to her getting less hungry and being able to carry out her tasks more efficiently. With the excess sugar out of her system, her brain fog slowly cleared, and she found herself getting more focused and motivated at work. Laura's fat slowly melted away. She lost 10 pounds in the first three weeks, and her steady fat loss continued as she regained her dream trim, fit figure which looked superb in anything she wore – whether it was a conservative shirt tucked into a skirt or a tasteful dinner gown. In the long-term, Laura confessed to feeling truly more alive, as she had even managed to cut down on the costs she incurred on purchasing her sugary treats – she hadn't only saved her career, she had preserved her health and her wallet too. Call that a three-pronged victory.

The sirtfood diet is not all about external looks, however, as Robert's story teaches us. Rob was a regular middle-aged guy in his forties who suffered from a severe case of depression. Robert was always on antidepressants and sedatives, and he relied heavily on these drugs to function as frequently as possible. A lot of times, Robert felt like giving up. At work and home, he tended to move mechanically as if in a daze, his mind clouded continuously with worry. Despite the potent sedatives that he used, on many nights, Robert would lie awake in bed, closing his eyes for long periods but unable to find sleep because of the thoughts raging in his mind. He was a brilliant man, but his mind was holding him down, mainly preventing him from achieving his full potential.

Robert's perpetual inactivity caused him to begin to gain weight over time. It wasn't like he was particularly concerned about that anyway; he had more significant problems going on in his head. However, he managed to discover the sirtfood diet, and in two weeks, Robert had managed to lose his first ten pounds of fat. That was not the most revolutionary change for him. For the first time in years, Robert managed to go through a week without having to battle his usual bouts of insomnia. Like magic, his self-esteem and personal happiness returned. His colleagues claimed they'd never seen Robert so happy to come to work. He seemed to have a glint in his eyes and a smile for everyone. Consequent to Robert's new diet, he found out that his general mood and his sleep pattern improved, he lost fat, especially around his abdominal region, and he felt himself look actually, fitter.

Here is Melanie's testimony, too, another beneficiary of the magic efficacy of the Sirtfood diet. Melanie was a middle-aged woman with lupus. She was held continuously down from the repeated pains and aches that the disease caused. This condition caused her to be quite inactive, causing her to put on quite a lot of unhealthy fat. Two weeks after she got on the sirtfood diet, her moods drastically improved, and her pains began to dissipate slowly. The polyphenols in the sirtfoods she was consuming activated her body's stress pathways causing her body to use up the fat and spurring the rejuvenation of her body's cells, including her diseased skin cells. Within two weeks, Melanie had managed to drop 11.5 pounds of fat, and her pains and aches were significantly relieved.

Now that we have examined some cases of individuals who have tried the sirtfood diet and experienced spectacular results, how about we back up these stories by looking at entire cultures and civilizations whose meals consist mainly of polyphenol-containing foods?

First, let's begin with Japan. When Japan is mentioned of all the countries on the Asian continent, so many people think of different things. Some set of people, what they instantly imagine is the clean streets and the lively, colorful culture. For some others, it is the discipline embedded in the culture of the Japanese that they are reminded of. It is the technological prowess for some others. Some people are told of the local Japanese cuisine, which consists of a lot of leafy vegetables. Whichever imagination you get first when you think of Japan, the truth is that the Japs are quite formidable people. There is, however, a subset of the Japanese who live in a province known as Okinawa. The people in this region have a local cuisine that consists almost exclusively of sirtfoods. The people in this region are rarely obese, have a relatively high life expectancy compared to most other areas of the world, and they are generally referred to as 'happy and lively.' The region is exclusively pulsating with life and excitement because the people don't stuff themselves with unhealthy junk food. Instead, they have grown up reaping the benefits of a diet that helps them to maintain fabulous moods and incredible, fit bodies.

The Native Mediterranean region is another region of the earth that is reputed for its healthy population and happy people. Native Mediterranean people have one of the lowest obesity and heart disease rates in the world. Their diets consist majorly of important sirtfoods such as extra virgin olive oil, wild leafy greens, nuts, berries, dates, and red wine. It is rare to find a person with a weight problem in this region, as they are known to live in perfect harmony with nature. It is not uncommon to find people living in cottages with lush gardens. Instead of counting calories and using manufactured drugs, the people of the Native Mediterranean Region simply choose to embrace nature by sticking to a healthy and nutritious diet.

So, there you have it. The sirtfood diet has been explaincd. Some of the people who have successfully used the diet to improve their physical and mental health have been highlighted. Entire cultures that have depended on sirtfood for generations upon generations for superb health and unrivaled happiness have been mentioned. Now, you may wonder: Exactly how effective is the sirtfood diet?

One of the most persuasive arguments in favor of sirtfoods is easy accessibility. With a trip to your regional grocery store, you can easily purchase the majority of the groceries that you need to prepare the foods in the sirtfood diet. The diet is affordable and easily accessible. A lot of less effective diets require you to purchase expensive supplements and scarce commodities, which make the practicability of these diets even less likely.

Because the diet aims to fill you up with enough healthy foods instead of stripping you of your necessary daily food supply, it is easier for you to stick to the diet in the long term, making it a beneficial weight-loss option. Combined with light exercise and great lifestyle habits, the sirtfood doesn't only help to reform your physical outlook but also has significant positive effects on your mental health.

Some of the trackable and significant effects of the sirtfood diet include:

- Fat loss
- Less risk of heart disease
- Fit, trim looks
- Increased energy and motivation
- Less hunger

- Improvement of physical strength.

Why are the selected food for the sirtfood diet so beneficial? The answer is simple and straightforward, as we have examined earlier. Sirtfoods have all been carefully chosen because they contain a specialized set of natural chemicals known as polyphenols. The polyphenols and the initial restriction of calories work together to activate the body's natural stress pathways, leading to the activation of the sirtuin genes. The sirtuin genes then direct the synthesis and deployment of natural body mechanisms that help to break down fat deposits to supply energy, rejuvenate and revitalize body cells and strengthen the body's natural immune system. The key factors that make the sirtfood diet so beneficial are the polyphenols in the foods and the calorie-restricting technique employed at the beginning of the diet.

Which foods are allowed to be consumed by someone going through the sirtfood diet? There are a variety of foods that contain the necessary polyphenols that can help activate the sirtuin genes in the body when eaten in appropriate quantities. Fruits, vegetables, fish, and other plant-based foods have been touted for years as the keys to weight loss and good health. While most of these foods contain essential nutrients such as vitamins, minerals, and proteins needed for disease prevention and optimal health, more often than not, they do not play direct roles in weight loss.

For a food-select to be allowed into a sirtfood diet, such food recipes must not contradict the functioning of the sirtfoods. This means that most plant-based foods, fresh fruits and vegetables, and fish are allowed. However, there are a couple of specific foods that form the core of the sirtfood diet. These foods and their active polyphenols include:

Sirtfood	**Active Polyphenol**
Arugula	Quercetin, Kaempferol
Buckwheat	Rutin
Capers	Kaempferol, Quercetin
Celery	Apigenin, Luteolin
Chilies	Luteolin, Myricetin

Cocoa	Epicatechin
Coffee	Caffeic Acid
Extra virgin olive oil	Oleuropein, hyroxytyrosol
Garlic	Myricetin, Ajoene
Green tea	Epicallocatechin gallate
Kale	Kaempferol, Quercetin
Medjool dates	Caffeic-acid, Gallic acid
Parsley	Apigenin, Myricetin
Red endive	Luteolin
Red onion	Quercetin
Red wine	Resveratrol
Soy	Formononentin
Strawberries	Fisetin
Turmeric	Curcumin
Walnuts	Gallic acid

If you hope to achieve any consistent results with the sirtfood diet, it is also critical that you avoid some foods altogether. The foods in question are going to affect the efficiency of the action of the sirtuin genes and work against your progress. These foods include:

Alcohols: Except for red wine, you need to steer clear of all kinds of alcoholic drinks as you take a step to begin your sirtfood diet journey. Whiskey, brandy, rum, vodka, beer, scotch, tequila, and martinis need to be laid off. Gently adopt the sophisticated practice of drinking red wine instead.

Saturated fats: Foods that contain red meat, hot dogs, sausages, and such like that contain saturated fats should be avoided if you hope for optimal results from the sirtfood diet.

Refined carbohydrates and processed sugar: Foods in this group have little fiber, and the body finds it difficult to digest them. The sugar tends to go straight into the bloodstream as glucose, raising the levels of insulin, the hormone that aids in controlling blood sugar. The secretion of insulin, in turn, leads to the inefficient breakdown of stored fats. This is why consistent consumption of processed sugar leads to the accumulation of fats in the body. So, if your body is trying to get rid of your excess fat stores and you keep piling up the fat even more, then you would be rendering the activities of the polyphenols in the sirtfoods ineffective. Foods such as potato chips, French fries, hash brownies, white bread, pasta, and crackers need to be avoided too.

Sugary snacks such as candy, ice cream, pastries, cakes, cookies, and muffins also need to be actively avoided. And I guess you know why this is the case? Yes, you're right- high content of processed sugar. Still on trying to cut down on your sugar consumption, avoiding sweetened drinks such as soda and fruit juices is also important for your enhanced progress with the sirtfood diet.

However, it is an all gloom, all doom situation. You still get to relish coffee, dark chocolate, and of course, red wine as a regular part of your diet while doing your body a great deal of good.

Sirtfoods stay atop unchallenged.

We have extensively gone over the mode of action of sirtfoods and the foods that possess the ability to activate the sirtuin genes. However, what exactly gives sirtfoods the edge over other forms of dieting out there? The simple answers are sustainability and multiple positive effects.

First, very significant among the most critical downsides of almost all dieting programs around the world is the problem of calorie restriction. Most diets work based on instructing people to eat certain foods in very strict rations while telling them to stay completely away from almost all the foods they used to love previously. This is placing two enormous strains on the individual all at once. Not only do they have to let go of their favorite sugary junk food that they've probably been hooked on for years, but these individuals also have to eat new, rather bland food in minimal quantities that end up making them famished. And far from helping matters is the fact that they also have to do that for the rest of their life? How does this plan sound? Utterly ridiculous, you think? Yeah, maybe a more cynical synonym would have looked better. The sad truth is that that's what a lot of dietitians out them expect patients to abide by.

However, forcing people to give up their sugary treats and eat vegetables twice a day while frantically calculating their calorie intake and freaking out when they 'mistakenly' eat a candy bar is not a sustainable way to build a healthy lifestyle. The sirtfood diet is characteristic of encouraging people to eat reasonable portions of healthy food. Sure, in phase 1, the calorie intake per day is restricted to ensure the activation of the Sirtuin genes. Still, once that phase is over, participants can go back to eating stable, healthy meals without the fear of exceeding any constraining calorie restrictions. This technique helps people to stay satiated and energized, thereby reducing their cravings for the unhealthy foods they used to indulge in. So, the sirtfood diet is more sustainable and reduces the chances of a person relapsing back into their old unhealthy eating habit, and this makes it a very practical option over other diets.

The fact that the sirtfood diet promotes the consumption of healthier food rather than the consumption of less food altogether makes it a fantastic contributor to the strength of an individual's immune system. The human immune system is immensely influenced by the quality of the food that an individual eats. Nutritious food substances such as those that make up the sirtfood diet contain natural chemical substances that aid the body's natural defense system. When these food substances are consumed in ample amounts that ensure satiety, they contribute a lot of helpful natural chemical substances to the body, thereby helping to reduce the chances of an individual developing a life-threatening ailment. Calorie-restricting diets, on the other hand, however, prevent the individual from consuming the amount of food that the body needs, thereby cutting down on the amount of significant natural chemicals that the immune system requires for optimal function.

Another point in favor of the sirtfood diet, as opposed to other diets, is the fact that it promotes the abundance of energy, strength, and muscle mass in an individual. As we've reiterated for the umpteenth time, the sirtfood diet encourages people to eat healthy food that promotes muscle gain and reduces the accumulation of fats. This simple phenomenon gives the sirtfood diet a significant edge over most other diets that focus mainly on restricting calorie intake. The fact that sirtfoods can be eaten until proper satiation is achieved means that people can stay energized and healthy to tackle their daily goals while gradually building up their muscle mass over time. Most of these other diets practically prevent people from eating enough at all, leading to drastic losses in muscle mass, dipping energy levels, and poor physical strength.

To wrap up this exhaustive expose on the sirtfoods and their functioning, let's look at a quick recap of how sirtfoods function and why they are so effective.

Sirtfoods, once again, are a group of foods that contain a specialized group of chemicals known as polyphenols. The polyphenols, in conjunction with the restriction of calories in the first phase of the diet, have the unique capability to activate a specialized stress pathway within the body system, which leads to the activation of the inducible sirtuin genes. The sirtuins, once activated, begin to direct a variety of important body-repair processes, which include the burning of fat deposits to provide ample energy for the body, the repair and rejuvenation of body cells, and the strengthening of the body's immune system. Important plant-based foods such as arugula, kale, turmeric, strawberries, red wine, cocoa, soy, red onions, and parsley form essential components of the sirtfood diet, mainly due to their sufficient polyphenol contents.

CHAPTER THREE

WELCOME TO THE FIRST LEAP

Having entirely understood what the sirtfood diet is, how it works, and the immense benefits that you can reap from this nutritional regimen, now, let's begin to explore the nitty-gritty of the implementation process gradually. How exactly are you supposed to eat the foods that make up the Sirtfood diet?

The first stage of the sirtfood is known as the first phase, or more commonly, 'Phase 1'. Step 1 refers basically to the first seven days of the sirtfood diet regimen. This first phase is the most intense of the sirtfood diet system as it is the only stage where you cannot consume above a specified number of calories. In the first three days of phase 1, the maximum permissible number of calories that can be consumed per day is one thousand. In the last four days, the maximum permitted number of consumable calories moves up to 1500. This phase is designed and aimed at helping you hit the ground running to activate your sirtuin genes. The restricted number of calories will aid in the activation of your body's stress pathways, which would eventually, together with the action other polyphenols in the sirtfoods, lead to the activation of the sirtuin genes.

At the conclusive end of the first phase, the average mass of fat that would be lost should be between 5 to 7 pounds. However, your body is most likely going to retain all of its muscle or even add up some more, so using a weighing scale to judge the progress of phase 2 might not be such a good idea. In synopsis, step 1 is the first seven days during which you are introduced to the sirtfood diet scheme.

How are you preparing for phase 1?

When you start on the sirtfood diet, you are preparing to begin a journey to a new kind of freedom and liberation – freedom from your self-imposed shackles of poor eating habits into a world where you have control over what goes in your body. To get started with the introductory phase, you will need to put a couple of things in place. These include:

A juicer: A lot of modern households already use a juicer in one way or the other on a fairly regular basis. The whole idea behind having a juicer is to help in the preparation of the sirtfood green juice, a natural concoction of herbs that would help detoxify your body and get you started on dissolving those fatty deposits. Since the aim of the juicer is to extract as much liquid as possible from vegetables, be sure to get one that is better equipped for the type of food products you would be putting in it.

Secondly, you would need to get familiar with your sirtfood menu and see where exactly you can get all these foods in your neighborhood. Depending on your city, you may be able to get all the sirtfoods you need in your local grocery store, or you may need to try shopping in the open market to get some of the vegetables and food items on the list. The point, however, is to get familiar with the foods that will be forming your new regimen and to figure out how you'd be sourcing these foods.

Also, you need to figure out a means of preserving the foods you'd be purchasing beforehand. If you have steady access to electricity and a refrigerator, it is advised that you shop for three days' worth of vegetable supplies at once, and store the veggies in your fridge for when you need to make your meals. After three days, you'd need another supply of vegetables. The three-day limit is set to prevent spoilage of the veggies, which would only affect the quality of your food and the rate of your development.

Likewise, you will have to learn how to prepare the foods you would make beforehand. The sirtfood menu features a variety of food options, so it's okay for you to select a few that you can confidently cook right away. As you progress in your journey in the diet, you will gradually learn how to cook more foods and expand your diet varieties.

Next on the to-do list on what to do to get started with the first stage of the Sirtfood diet is to plan your eating timetable. Your sirtfood green juice should be consumed three times per day in the first three days – once when you wake up, thirty minutes to one hour before any meal, and then two other times within the day. Look at your number of calories and plan out when you would be eating and what you would be eating on each day. This will make it an easy route for you to make these decisions when you finally begin your diet.

Journaling can be beneficial in your attempt to

stay steadfast and committed to your journey. This avails you room to keep a chronological record of your struggles and your victories as you go through the sirtfood diet. Journaling daily will not only motivate you to rise the next day and stick religiously to your diet, but it will also help you to remember how much you have given up to stay healthy and ginger you to keep going when the going gets tough.

Trying to use the scales to monitor your progress, especially so early into your dieting journey, is a bad idea. As has been repeatedly mentioned, the sirtfood diet helps you to burn fats as well as maintain and even build muscle mass. Consequently, as you gear up to begin phase 1 of your diet, try as much as possible to stay off the scales for the meantime and just focus on sticking to this wonderful dieting system.

Finally, get excited about the journey ahead. To accomplish this, it helps if you can figure out exactly why you are embarking on the sirtfood diet. Are you doing it to reduce your risk of contracting a dangerous life0threatening disease along the line? Are you doing it to enhance your career in the media or modeling industry? Are you doing it to improve your mental health and improve your moods, focus, and concentration? Whatever be your reason for wanting to make the crucial personal sacrifice of starting up the sirtfood diet, remind yourself that you are finally about to achieve those aims. Be excited that your life is about to experience a positive turn around.

Expectations for Phase 1

Manifestations come from being expectant.

No one receives a thing without being prepared to receive.

You may wonder – what exactly is Phase 1 going to entail, and what results can I expect to achieve after the first week of my diet? With great sacrifice, they say, comes great rewards. Phase 1 is going to be the most tasking phase of your diet, no doubt, but it will also be the phase that provides you with the most pleasantly surprising results. At the end of step 1, you can expect to lose between 5 to 7 pounds of weight in pure fat, as evidenced by the results of the cohort study carried out in London. You can also expect to experience enhanced mental clarity and focus, and a general feeling of lightness and agility.

Meanwhile, since phase 1 is going to be your stage of making the most critical sacrifices for future benefits, it also means you would probably have to deal with some discomfort during this phase. Although it isn't everybody who will most likely experience these signs, yet some participants in the diet have reported feelings of hunger, lethargy, slight irritability, and even intense cravings for junk food and sugary snacks and drinks during the first phase. It is believed that the restriction of the calories consumed by the participant in the early three days to one thousand calories, and to fifteen hundred calories in the last four days of phase one is responsible for these challenges. So, it not entirely one of those extreme discomforts. Pretty good, it is dependent on the type of individual.

Therefore, in the case of you feeling really hungry, tired, or extremely desirous of junk food during your first phase, being patient is all you need. Remember your reason for starting this, and renew your resolve to stay healthy while fighting for the dazzling life you've dreamed of every single day. Usually, in the final days of this phase, as your body gets used to the diet, you will feel your fatigue and tiredness slipping away. These feelings would become replaced by those of unusual strength, clarity, and agility. As you switch from one thousand calories to fifteen hundred calories per day, you will feel more satiated and energized too. Do you think it all ends there? You can be sure that your moods will generally improve also. From this point onwards, your journey becomes progressively easier.

Meal plan for Phase 1

Everything in life requires planning. Sometimes, it is not just about planning, but doing so adequately. More like the famous maxim, if you fail to plan, you plan to fail. The quest to be successful at anything at all begins on the verge of planning. This isn't different when it comes to keeping the body and health in their right shapes. It is, of course, the case for the first phase of the Sirtfood diet system.

For the first three days of the sirtfood diet, you will be expected to drink three sirtfood juices and eat one mail sirtfood meal per day. This combination helps you to keep the number of calories consumed just under one thousand. For the last four days of the first phase, however, you will be required to eat two main sirtfood meals and two sirtfood juices daily. This combination would sum up to about fifteen hundred calories, as has been previously highlighted.

As you may have probably predicted, the sirtfood green juice would be an essential part of your sirtfood diet in phase one and beyond. After water, this drink would constitute a significant percentage of your total fluid intake as you proceed with the sirtfood diet. Other fluids that you would be permitted to consume would include black coffee (i.e., without milk) and green tea. You should abstain from dairy during the first phase of the sirtfood diet as it contains active substances that may hamper the activation of the sirtuin genes.

Since the sirtfood green juice is so critical to the success of your sirtfood diet, let's examine precisely how to make the sirtfood green juice before delving into what your model meal plan should look like.

To prepare the sirtfood green juice, you'll need:

2.5 oz. kale

1 oz. arugula

0.25 oz. flat-leaf parsley

5.5 oz. celery stalks (with leaves)

0.5 medium green apple

1 in. ginger

Half of a lemon, squeezed or juiced.

0.5 tsp. matcha powder

Note that the matcha powder should only be included only in the first two juices of the day during the first three days of phase one. Specifically, between days 1 and 3, matcha should be added to both your early morning juice before breakfast, as well as the drink you'll be having by midmorning. Your third sirtfood juice of the day should, however, not contain matcha powder because the substance is caffeinated and may alter your sleep pattern if taken too late in the day. So, do not forget – no matcha for the last juice of the day between days 1 and 3.

For the final four days of phase one, however, it is okay to put matcha powder in the two sirtfood juices you'll be drinking daily. This is because you'd have completed your daily required sirtfood juice intake by midday, provided you follow the laid-down guidelines religiously.

So, now that you know both the ingredients and the sirtfood juice rules let's get into the nitty-gritty of making this wholesome drink.

First of all, mix your veggies in the juicer. In other words, your arugula, kale, and parsley should be loaded into the juicer. Ensure to extract as much fluid as possible from these greens so that you get maximum value for your time, effort, and money. After the juicing process, you should have obtained about a quarter of a cup of veggie juice, which is ready for use.

The next step is to lead your apples, ginger, and celery into the juicer and extract the fluid from those too. Add this new mixture to the one obtained in the first step.

Then, peel your lemon, cut it in half, and squeeze out the juice. If you feel that your squeezing is not efficient enough, you can use the juicer instead. After adding the lemon juice to your mixture, you should have about a cup of juice ready.

Pour out a small portion of your juice and add in your half teaspoon of matcha powder. Ensure that the matcha dissolves appropriately in the sauce, and then pour the matcha-containing juice into the rest of the sauce.

Stir your juice properly, and you may add a little water to adjust the taste if you like. Enjoy the immaculate taste of good health! It doesn't get better than that.

Having gotten a good feel and grasp of how to

make your sirtfood green juice, the next line of action is to design a workable meal plan that would allow you to access a variety of sirtfoods that will aid your progress in phase 1. Remember that in each day for your first three days, you must drink a cup of sirtfood green juice thrice, and eat a sirtfood main meal once. For the remaining four days of Phase 1, it's two sirtfood juices and two main meals to give fifteen hundred calories.

Let's break the meal plan down now.

Day 1: Sirtfood green juice – 3 times

Main meal – 1 time

Meal idea: Stir-fried Asian shrimp, buckwheat noodles and dark chocolate (85% cocoa)

Vegan option: Sesame glazed tofu, miso, ginger, chili, stir-fried greens, and dark chocolate (85% cocoa).

Day 2: Sirtfood green juice – 3 times

Main meal: 1 time

Meal idea: Aromatic chicken breast, kale, red onions, tomato, and chili salsa

Vegan option: Kale, red onion dal, and buckwheat.

Day 3: Sirtfood green juice – 3 times

Main meal: 1 time

Meal idea: Turkey escalope, capers, sage, parsley, cauliflower, and dark chocolate.

Vegan option: Baked tofu, cauliflower, and dark chocolate.

From day four onwards, you can eat ½ oz. Dark chocolate once a day, preferably alongside one meal.

Day 4: Sirtfood green juice – 2 times

Main meal: 2 times

Meal 1: Sirt muesli

Meal 2: Salmon fillet, endive, arugula, and celery salad.

Vegan option 1: Sirt muesli

Vegan option 2: Tuscan bean stew.

Day 5: Sirtfood green juice – 2 times

Main meal: 2 times

Meal 1 (Vegan and regular diets): Sirt super salad.

Meal 2 (regular diet): Grilled beef, red wine, onion rings, garlic, kale, and roasted potatoes.

Meal 2 (Vegan diet): Kidney bean mole and baked potatoes.

Day 6: Sirtfood green juice – 2 times

Main meal: 2 times

Meal 1: Sirtfood omelet

Meal 2: Baked chicken breast, parsley pesto, red onion salad.

Vegan option 1: Waldorf salad.

Vegan option 2: Roasted eggplants, walnuts, parsley pesto, and tomato salad.

Day 7: Sirtfood green juice – 2 times

Main meal: 2 times

Meal 1: Strawberry buckwheat salad

Meal 2: Baked cod marinated in miso, sesame, and stir-fried greens

Vegan option 1: Strawberry buckwheat salad.

Vegan option 2: Buckwheat noodles in miso broth, tofu, celery, and kale.

CHAPTER FOUR

THE SECOND LEAP AFTER THE FIRST

What is Phase 2?

In the previous chapter, we extensively described what Phase 1 of the sirtfood diet is about. Now, the journey can only get more and more enjoyable. Since life in itself doesn't stop at just taking only the first leap, achieving a hundred percent result with the Sirtfood diet requires a continuous effort and commitment to the set plan. After successfully completing the early seven days of the sirtfood diet, then you would be starting Phase 2 on the 8th day. Phase 2 simply refers to two weeks after the first seven days of the sirtfood diet. Phase two is a nutrient-packed 14-day period that allows you to raise your calorie consumption while integrating the sirtfood diet into your usual daily routine.

In phase 2 of the sirtfood diet, it is expected that your fat loss would record more improvement and progress. As step 2 progresses, if you stick steadfastly to your diet, you are likely to find yourself getting slimmer and feeling even more energized and pumped to tackle your daily tasks. While on course with this second phase, you would be eating three times a day, meaning that issues of hunger, fatigue, and irritability due to restriction of calories should not be a problem here. Even though it is advised that you eat thrice, yet, we recommend that you do not over-eat. Eat till you feel full and satisfied, and then stop. Satisfaction and sustainability are the hallmarks of phase 2. More important, this phase, if handled well, will help you integrate the sirtfood diet into your lifestyle, rather than merely being synthetic.

Girding up for the second leap

There are petty pointers that you harmonize and probably start implementing right from your first phase to help you coast through the second phase of the sirtfood diet successfully. Only the first leap will convince you. These tips include:

Rise early: As we have mentioned in the previous chapter, the sirtfood green juice remains a crucial and critical part of your diet. To ensure that you maximize the benefits of this power drink, you must drink it thirty minutes to one hour before having your main breakfast. You can regard this as the pre-breakfast diet. When you wake up early each day, you will be encouraged to drink your sirtfood green juice, get a little workout done, and get ready for work before finally eating your healthy sirtfood breakfast. The combination of the sirtfood meal and the sirtfood green juice will help fill you up and energized to maximize your day, while of course, helping you to melt away those fat deposits along the way.

Eat dinner early: Whether you are on a diet or not, medical experts generally advise against later night eating. It is healthier to eat your dinner early, between 6 PM and 7 PM, and then get a little rest before retiring to bed. So, instead of working late and wolfing down a heavy dinner in bed at 11 PM, try to take a break, eat your healthy dinner, and then get back to handling the rest of your work. It helps if you are done with your work at least one hour before bed so that you can allow your body to calm down before you sleep gradually. To ensure the optimal success of the sirtfood diet, you should get an average of 7 -8 hours of sleep per night. If you are extremely busy, try to get at least 6 hours of sleep every night. That will help the nutrients in the food repair and rejuvenate your body cells, which will make you healthier, stronger, and well-built. Sleeping early also makes you focused and energized when you wake up to tackle the challenges of the next day.

Eat balanced, measured potions: It is essential to strike a balance in the quantity of food you would be eating. Overeat, and you would be overloading your body with calories. You may think: "But the aim is to get as much of the important chemicals as possible!". Yes, you want to have as many polyphenols as healthily possible into your system, but over-eating can cause constipation and affect the action of the sirtuins in your body. So, eat till you are satiated, and then stop. Since you will be eating three meals per day in the second phase, there is no need for you to overload yourself at any time. Eat till you feel reasonably satisfied, get to work, and then eat another meal later. This is not to mean that you should go hungry. However, you don't have to overload yourself to the point of lethargy either. Let your appetite guide you and stay energized and focused.

Remember that healthy diets are those kept within measures.

Drink your sirtfood juice once: As you already know now, the sirtfood juice is an excellent source of nutrients and polyphenols for activating your sirtuin genes. However, as you progress with the diet and eat more food daily, you are required to gradually begin to slow down your consumption of the sirtfood green juice. You will recall that in Phase 1, the sirtfood green juice was recommended to be consumed thrice per day alongside one meal for the first three days. In the last four days of phase 1, the daily recommended intake of the sirtfood green juice reduces to two cups, and you become required to eat two meals per day. Once you transition into phase 2 of your diet plan, however, things change. You can now eat three meals per day, meaning you can get an optimum supply of your nutrients from your food, also indicating that an intense calorie restriction is no longer necessary. For this reason, once phase 2 begins, you should only consume your sirtfood green juice only once a day – and that's very early in the morning, thirty minutes to one hour before your main breakfast as usual.

Apart from the sirtfood green juice, you can still drink a couple of liquids in phase 2 of the diet. These liquids include water, flavored water, black coffee, and green tea. You may also consume red wine up to three times a week as soon as you commence phase 2.

Expectations for Phase 2

In phase 2, your weight loss journey is due to continue. The amount of fat that would be eradicated in this phase would vary from one individual to another. However, it is not unconventional for people to lose up to 10 more pounds in pure fat in this phase. As we continuously advise, do not try to judge the success of your dieting efforts by checking a weighing scale every morning. The diet is aimed at helping you burn fat and improve your muscle mass. Therefore, while losing fat, your muscle cells may be actively dividing, thereby helping you to increase your muscle mass. One way by which you can track your fat loss rate isn't by periodically looking up your body in the mirror but by merely checking the fit of your clothes, or asking for a few trusted opinions.

By its design, the second phase is meant to come with enhanced focus and vitality. The active components of the sirtfoods will continue to keep your sirtuin genes activated, leading to feelings of enhanced mental clarity and boosted concentration. The consumption of the foods contained in the sirtfood diet helps to rejuvenate your brain cells, thereby helping to improve brainpower.

If you were addicted to junk food and sugary products before staring at the sirtfood diet, phase 2 is no doubt the stage where your cravings begin to lessen considerably. This is because you would be having three healthy meals per day, and a nutrient-packed cup of green juice with which to start your day. Your body would always feel satiated, and that urge to dash across the street to grab a burger and a soda just won't be there since you would not be feeling hungry in the first place.

Just as we have highlighted earlier in this book, the consumption of unhealthy food leads to the accumulation of fat deposits in the body. When you consume a lot of processed sugar regularly, the sugar will gain easy access to your bloodstream, increasing your blood sugar levels, and by extension, your insulin levels. Once your insulin levels pass a certain safe threshold, the natural burning of fats in the body is suppressed, and you begin to trend towards obesity. With obesity comes a high likelihood of heart disease since the fats would make it compulsory for the heart to pump blood at unhealthily high pressure. In some cases, the fat deposits may even block critical blood vessels within the body, which can lead to falling unconscious and even death. However, with this second phase in place, there is a high chance that your susceptibility to debilitating diseases will be significantly reduced.

Meal Plan for Phase 2

First and foremost, note that the rule is still the same for sirtfood juice throughout the fourteen days. Secondly, your eating is kept at three standard meals a day – breakfast, lunch, and dinner. These meals will provide your body with the necessary calories and nutrients it needs to stay energized and satiated while eradicating unhealthy fat deposits and repairing your body's cells. In phase 2, carefully selected sirtfood snacks may also be introduced, and they may be consumed once or twice per day. The sirtfood snacks can mainly come in handy when you are in a position where you cannot have a standard meal right away. So instead of violating your diet's rules and eating unhealthy junk, you can simply have a healthy sirtfood snack, pending the time you can eat a standard meal. Sirtfood snacks can be particularly great for long meetings, flights, and long road travels, shopping, and other related circumstances.

One final reminder, however, the sirtfood diet

works best when the foods digest and get the chance to start working before you go to bed, so your dinner should not exceed 7 PM.

Breakfast Options

The foods in this section may be eaten at 7-day intervals. Depending on your preferences and schedule, however, you can modify this suggestion to fit your lifestyle. Meal option one may be eaten on the eighth day of your diet and the 15th day, for instance. Meal 2, on the other hand, maybe eaten on day 9 of the diet and day 16. More important, ensure that the food is varied as possible while as many meals are eaten before consuming the same food again.

The breakfast options include:

Sirtfood smoothie

Sirt muesli

Yogurt, berries, walnut and dark chocolate

Spicy scrambled eggs

Mushroom/ tofu scramble

Buckwheat pancakes, walnuts, strawberries and chocolate

Sirtfood omelet.

Lunch options

Just as instructed for the breakfast options, the lunch options may also be eaten once a week, preferably on a specific day of the week to help you vary your diet and find your new feeding regimen interesting. Lunch options include:

Sirt chicken salad.

Waldorf salad – apples, walnuts, celery, and mayonnaise.

Sirt tuna salad.

Strawberry buckwheat salad.

Buckwheat pasta salad.

Tofu and shiitake mushroom soup

Whole wheat leavened bread.

Dinner options

Foods that may be eaten for dinner during phase 2 of the sirtfood diet include:

Stir-fry shrimp and buckwheat noodles.

Tuscan bean stew.

Potatoes, kale, curry, and chicken.

Kale, red onions and buckwheat

Sirt chili con carne

Kidney bean mole and baked potatoes

Sirtfood pizza.

CHAPTER FIVE

GETTING STARTED WITH YOUR SHOPPING LIST

The previous chapters have been dedicated to unraveling what the Sirtfood diet entails. It is only progressive if you take another step towards actualizing your dreams of morphing into your dream figure and improving your overall physical and mental health. In this chapter, we would be looking at the twenty essential food items that make up the core of the sirtfood diet, why these foods are so crucial to the journey you are about to undertake, and how much these foods are likely to cost. As we journey through this chapter, you would notice that a lot of the core sirtfoods are vegetables. Hence, you can easily purchase them at the produce section of your local grocery store. Where possible, you can buy these food items in their natural state instead of in their processed form. However, some of these foods are going to have to be processed, so we would be looking at the best possible brands whose composition would allow you to achieve the most desired results for your dieting efforts.

The foods select in this section do not form an exhaustive list of foods that have the power to activate the dominant sirtuin genes. There are several other foods, most of them, fruits, vegetables, and whole grains that have considerable levels of polyphenols, which have significant effects on weight loss and cell rejuvenation too. However, the top twenty sirtfoods have been proven by research to be the essential sirtfoods discovered to date. Hence, we would be closely examining each of these sirtfoods in this chapter. You would be using most of these foods to prepare your meals during and beyond phase 1 and phase 2. As a result, we would be examining the prices of these food products, their health benefits, and recommended brands in cases where you can get pure organic fresh produce.

Berries come first on the list. They are part of the top 20 sirtfoods, and they contain enormous amounts of Fisetin, an important polyphenol that has important antioxidative and anti-carcinogenic properties. While strawberries are core sirtfoods, other berries also contain varying concentrations of other vital polyphenols and can be ingested as a part of the sirtfood diet too. Blackberries, blackcurrants, blueberries, and raspberries are not essential sirtfoods, but they can help significantly on your journey to weight loss. Their efficacy also spans through the enhancement of physical and mental health.

Nuts are another group of foods with one essential representative in the top twenty sirtfoods, but with other members packing different levels of primary polyphenols. Walnuts are perfect examples of core sirtfoods, due to the high concentration of Gallic acid in them. Chestnuts, pecans, pistachios, and peanuts, however, also contain other essential biochemicals that have been proven to significantly help in fat loss as well as lowering the risk of chronic diseases. You have to be intentional when it comes to consuming nuts. This is because some individuals have been found to have allergies for nuts. Peanut allergies are particularly common in the United States.

Whole grains are also important foods whose

immense health impacts extend to helping individuals lose unhealthy fat deposits and prevent the development of chronic diseases. Whole grains contain a high content of sirtuin activators; however, once the grains are processed and become white, most of the essential nutrients get stripped off during the refining process. Therefore, processed grains are a good source of pure carbohydrate, which you don't want too much of if you are trying to lose weight. If you stick with whole grains such as unprocessed wheat and rice, you are likely to reap a lot of important health benefits than if you choose the processed versions of these foods. The good news is that if you are trying to stay gluten-free, you can find the perfect gluten-free whole grain options for you at most grocery stores near you. If you are also looking forward to indulging in a healthy snack every now and then, popcorn serves a great way to keep you filled while ensuring that you do not fill your body up with unhealthy carbohydrates.

Now, let's get into your shopping list for the top twenty sirtfoods that you would have to purchase as basics once you're ready to start up your sirtfood diet. Trust me; the first item is an interesting one.

Dark Chocolate: Chocolate has always been an

all-time favorite among adults and children alike all over the world. There are quite a number of chocolate types, however. So that you know, chocolate is usually classified based on the percentage of the various constituents it contains. Milk chocolate bars are quite popular in the US and other parts of the world. Still, as we mentioned earlier, the aim is to keep your milk consumption as low as possible, since milk potentially interferes with the activation of the sirtuin genes. The specific type of chocolate that is best for this diet is dark chocolate. This chocolate variety should contain an optimal 85% of cocoa, with the remaining 15%$ being a mix of other constituents. Dark chocolate's extremely high cocoa content makes it a rich source of the polyphenol Epicatechin, which functions in helping to lower blood pressure by removing any fatty instructions in the body's vascular system.

As we have reviewed earlier, one of the major causes of high blood pressure is the presence of numerous fatty deposits in the major blood vessels of the body. This condition puts the heart under too much pressure to pump blood to all parts of the body. By helping to clear the fat deposits in the blood vessels, the long-term consumption of Epicatechin in dark cocoa helps to improve cardiac health and vascular function in the body. Epicatechin has also been proven to boost cognitive function greatly. The polyphenol can help boost cell division rate and slow down cell damage in the brain, thereby helping to improve an individual's cognitive abilities, including memory and information processing functions. Similarly, cocoa has been proven to aid skin protection from the harmful ultraviolet rays of the sun.

While shopping for your dark chocolate, it is of high essence to look out for brands that have undergone an alkalization process known as 'dutching.' Dutching method is used mainly for preserving the chocolate, but it affects the concentration of the polyphenols that we need in our chocolate. Dark chocolate contains a low sugar content, meaning that it would help you relish the inimitable taste of chocolate without flooding your body with unhealthy processed sugar. Dark chocolate also contains fewer additives and preservatives that can affect the positive effects of the polyphenols contained in it. Including dark chocolate as a regular feature in your diet can help curb your sugar cravings and boost the endorphin and serotonin levels in your brain, thereby helping to significantly improve your mood, eradicate irritability and fatigue, and help you stay focused and motivated for a more extended period.

There is a brand of recommended dark chocolates that you can shop online or in a local store near you. These include Endangered Species Dark Chocolate, Alter Eco Dark Chocolate, Taza Dark Chocolate, and Lindt Dark Chocolate. You can obtain packs of these dark chocolate brands from between $15 to $40, depending on your outlet and preferred brand.

Red Wine: A lot of people who know a thing or two about the sirtfood diet will tell you that the inclusion of red wine in this diet is one of its most enjoyable parts. Red wine contains a considerably high amount of antioxidants and anti-inflammatory agents. Red wine contains high concentrations of resveratrol, one of the first polyphenols ever discovered. Resvcratrol has also been proven to promote healthy aging and prevent various types of cancers. Red wine's high resveratrol content enables it to help prevent the formation of blood clots within your blood vessels. As some individuals age, due to the lack of necessary thinning agents in their blood, possibly due to an unhealthy diet or due to genetics, blood clots may form within their vascular system. If these blood clots happen to block blood flow to a critical organ like the brain, the person might die a sudden, painful death. A glass of red wine a day, possibly with your last meal of the day can be a very significant addition to your diet.

Recommended brands of red wine include the Oak Leaf Vineyards Cabernet Sauvignon Red Wine and the Franzia Cabernet Red Wine. You can obtain a bottle of these wines under $20 at a local store near you.

Red Onions: While onions have a reputation for being one of the world's most popular food flavoring agents, not much is usually discussed about this superfood's incredible immune-system boosting properties. Red onions have high concentrations of the polyphenol Quercetin, antioxidants, and Vitamin C, making it a powerhouse capable of preventing a wide variety of diseases from cancers to heart diseases. The antioxidants in red onions okay pivotal roles in reversing the effects of free radicals. Should you be anxious to know, free radicals can lead to damaged cells and accelerated aging. Onions may also play important roles in accelerating the healing of internal and external wounds such as ulcers. Red onions generally have a low amount of calories, making them a valuable addition to the sirtfood diet. You can purchase fresh red onions from your local produce store at under $2 per pound.

Green Tea: Tea is one of the most popular beverages in the world. In ancient Asian civilizations, tea was considered a culturally significant drink because of its recognized healing and calming properties. Green tea contains a specific polyphenol compound known as Epicatechin gallate. This polyphenol plays a vital role in weight loss. If you remember the process for making the sirtfood green juice, you'd recall that matcha (a form of green tea) was required to be included in the juice because of its superior fat-burning abilities. Green tea contains a superb concentration of antioxidants that play huge roles in helping to prevent the body's cells from the damage caused by free radicals. Green tea has also proven to possess the ability to improve metabolic rates, thereby enhancing the rate of digestion and absorption of food into the body. High metabolic rates would help get you energized faster and will keep you going for longer.

Research has also shown that Green tea is effective at preventing and mitigating inflammations in the body. Green tea's polyphenol content also enables it to play a crucial role in the prevention of heart and brain disorders. By helping to burn the fat deposits within the body rapidly, green tea can help prevent heart diseases in the long-term. By aiding the rapid repair and rejuvenation of the brain cells, green tea helps to promote long-term brain health and helps to boost cognitive functions in the short term.

Recommended brands of green tea include Celestial Seasonings Green Tea and Great Value Green Tea. You can buy most green tea packs between $10 to $15 in the US.

Coffee: Once again, we have another popular American beverage. Coffee has grown to become an indispensable part of the lives of billions of people around the world, from professionals in the corporate world to entrepreneurs and academics. Coffee is renowned for its stimulating and relaxing abilities and is usually consumed in the morning and early in the afternoon. The chances that you drink coffee, at least on a fairly regular basis already, is quite high, considering how effectively it works. However, as you opt in to the sirtfood diet, you must understand that you would now be required to take your coffee black (i.e., without milk and preferably without processed sugar). Black coffee enables you to experience the distinctive flavor of coffee in all its glory and offers your body astonishing health benefits.

Coffee has been known to give the body a sharp energy boost, as it helps its consumers to stay alert early in the day. Statistics have also shown that coffee significantly improves brain function in both the short-term and long-term run. Caffeic acid is the active polyphenol on coffee, and it is a fact this amazing biochemical is capable of burning fat deposits in the body, thereby helping to lower the risk of a variety of diseases extending from Type 2 diabetes to heart disease. Coffee's brain stimulating properties make it a great preventive food against cognitive deficiencies such as Alzheimer's, dementia, and Parkinson's disease. The regular consumption of coffee also proves to help in the fight against cancer depression and liver damage.

Recommended coffee brands that you need to start your diet include Folger's Classic Roast, Maxwell House Light Roast, and McCafe Light Roast Coffee. These coffee brands can be bought online or at any local store near you between $15 to $20.

Arugula: Arugula is one of the most potent green vegetables in the sirtfood diet, and is undoubtedly one of the most nutritionally beneficial foods among the top twenty sirtfoods. For a fact, it has been confirmed to help boost weight loss due to the presence of the essential polyphenols – quercetin and Kaempferol that are present in this vegetable. Arugula contains a variety of essential nutrients ranging from Calcium, which can help strengthen bones and teeth. It also contains Potassium, which aids in nervous coordination and proper functioning of the brain function. Folate, which is highly crucial for the development of fetal in pregnant women, is equally found in Arugula. So also is Vitamin C and K, which help to boost the power of the immune system and in blood coagulation to prevent bleeding in the case of an injury.

Arugula's important polyphenols play significant roles in the repair and rejuvenation of damaged brain cells. This helps to prevent the brains of aging people from rapid dopamine decline. Arugula also boosts bone strength, helps remove harmful toxins from the body system, and has been found to exhibit important anti-inflammatory effects in the body. Since arugula is a green vegetable, it is best to buy it fresh and unpackaged. You can get a pound of arugula from your local grocery's produce section for less than $15 per pound.

Buckwheat: Buckwheat is an important core sirtfood of Asian origins that features the polyphenol Rutin. To a much-coveted degree, the buckwheat can significantly lower the body's cholesterol levels, thereby helping to decrease the risk of heart disease in the long term. It is equally very renowned for the pivotal roles that it plays in helping to lower the blood sugar level. It combines this with the ability to initiate a decrease in the body's insulin levels. The result of this is a direct reduction in the risk of type 2 diabetes and making the fat loss process significantly easier. Buckwheat is rich in dietary fibers, which aid digestion and prevent constipation and flatulence. Because of its richness in proteins, it can help play very germane roles in the prevention and retardation of cancerous growths.

Recommended buckwheat brands include Arrowhead Mills Organic Buckwheat Groats and Bob's Red Mill Organic Buckwheat Groats. You can get a can of buckwheat groats between $10 and $15, depending on your location.

Capers: A caper is a flower-bud gotten from a particular shrub that is said to have originated from Southern Europe. Capers contain the important polyphenols Rutin and Quercetin, which both aid in cell rejuvenation and the prevention of internal inflammations within the body system. Capers have significant percentages of antioxidants that play vital roles in counteracting the oxidative effects of free radicals on the body's organs. Free radicals may be generated by eating some of the more harmful conventional foods we eat, and they may hasten the aging process, leading to the breakdown of essential tissues and organs, and hasten the onset of chronic diseases. Antioxidants in capers, however, play significant roles in helping to wipe out these free radicals. Capers also promote the smooth circulation of blood in the body. When fat deposits block blood vessels, the heart would need to pump blood at a higher pressure. Most times, this often leads to what's popularly known as hypertension. In some situations, the blood supply to important extremities may be cut off. When this is the case, eating capers and other sirtfood greens is one tested and trusted way to constantly clean up the vascular system and prevent blood circulation problems. Capers are also loaded with essential macronutrients such as Calcium which supports strong bones and teeth, Iron that promotes the retention of oxygen in the blood, copper which catalyzes many of the body's natural biochemical processes, and sodium which is critical to the proper functioning of the body's nervous system.

Capers have also been discovered to help in mitigating conditions related to indigestion and constipation. This is because capers have relatively high fiber content, and fibers can smoothen and quicken body metabolism. The regular consumption of capers may also help prevent rheumatism, diabetes, low blood sugar, and skin problems.

If you can obtain fresh capers in your local store, then that would be wonderful. However, if you can't, you can count on trusted brands such as Paesana Non-Pareil Capers, and San Antonio Non-Pareil Capers. The 32oz. Packs of both sell for less than $20.

Celery: Celery is a vegetable that has become an integral part of most American diets; therefore, it is hardly a food that needs a lot of introduction. Celery, when consumed together with its leaves, is quite rich in a lot of essential vitamins and minerals. Apart from helping with the activation of your sirtuin genes, and by extension, weight loss and optimum well-being, celery furnishes your body with Vitamin K. Of course, you know, Vitamin K helps your blood clot properly in the case of wounds. Celery also is a source of Potassium (aids in nervous coordination); Vitamin A (improves the eyesight); and Folate that is exceptive to the growth and development of fetuses in the womb.

Like the others, Celery is rich in antioxidative and anti-inflammatory properties and can help aid digestion. It is advisable to purchase this vegetable from the fresh produce section of your local grocery store. You can buy Celery at under $3/kilogram.

Chilies: Chilies are another spicy American favorite. Several fast-food joints sell thousands of plates of chili-based foods around the country. However, we still recommend that you cook your chili-based meals at home, as we assure you that they can prevent and manage inflammation while helping to relieve the body from pains. Chilies can also help to improve cardiac health and then lessen the chances of you contracting a cardiovascular disease down the line by helping to rid the body of unnecessary fat deposits. Also, they help to clear congestion, boost immunity, and of course, burn off fats.

You can purchase fresh chili from the produce section of your local grocery. Prices usually range between $2 -$3 per kilogram.

Extra Virgin Olive Oil: This essential food product is one of the key constituents of the native Mediterranean diet that makes people from that region so healthy and physically fit. Extra virgin olive oil has a great capacity to burn off fats from the body, thereby helping to reduce the risk of heart disease significantly and helping you to achieve your dream body. Extra virgin olive oil plays important roles in helping to improve blood circulation and removing vascular debris, thereby reducing the chances of a stroke. A stroke occurs when blood flow to the brain is interrupted. However, when extra virgin olive oil is consumed regularly alongside other healthy sirtfoods, most of the vascular debris in your blood vessels would be regularly flushed out. When this happens, they help to keep you healthy for a longer time. Due to its spectacular fat-burning abilities, extra virgin olive oil also helps to lower the risk of Type 2 diabetes.

Extra virgin olive oil is active against cancer-causing agents, and its cell rejuvenation capabilities make it active in the prevention of cognitive decline and the enhancement of memory.

Recommended extra virgin olive oil brands include Great Value 1005 Extra Virgin Olive Oil and Pompeian Smooth Extra Virgin Olive Oil. Both can be gotten between $5 - $10 per bottle.

Garlic: Garlic is a member of the allium family, and it consists of leeks, shallot, and onions. Garlic contains a high concentration of essential vitamins and minerals that aid the proper functioning of the human body. Garlic is loaded with Vitamin C, which boosts the body's immunity and promotes the healing of wounds and Fibers, which helps with digestion and regent constipation. Due to its ability to efficiently burn up the body's fat deposits without affecting muscle gain, garlic is highly potential for bodybuilding and weight loss. More significantly, its ability to remove harmful cholesterol from the body is reputable for its role in lowering the risk of heart disease in the long terms run. Garlic, noteworthily, also helps to reduce the rate of cell death and promotes the rejuvenation and repair of damaged cells, thereby helping to slow down the aging process.

It is best to buy fresh organic garlic from the produce section of your grocery store. Fresh garlic prices should range around $4 per pound. But then, you can also get a 9.5-ounce tin of minced garlic for about $4 too.

Kale: Kale is popularly referred to as a superfood by most new-age nutritionists, and it is indeed one of the most richly endowed vegetables available today. Kale has a high concentration if the polyphenols Quercetin and Kaempferol, thereby helping to burn up body fats and boost natural immunity. Kale's immunity-boosting properties are compounded even further by the presence of Vitamin C, which accelerates the healing of wounds and the presence of antioxidants that play vital roles in counteracting the nocuous effects of free radicals on the body. Kale's high Vitamin K content promotes the clotting of blood, and its ability to remove cholesterol from the body. As a matter of fact, it helps to lessen the chances of heart disease in the long run. Kale has also been reported to contain significant levels of Vitamin A, Vitamin B6, Manganese, Calcium, Copper, Potassium, and Magnesium.

The presence of the biochemical Lutein and Zeaxanthin help in conjunction with kale's significant Vitamin A and Beta carotene to greatly improve eye-sight, and prevent eye disorders in the long term. Like all leafy vegetables, it is advisable to purchase kale fresh from the organic produce section of your local grocery. At $1 per pound, kale is one hell of an affordable magic health potion.

Medjool dates: Medjool dates are sweeter, larger, and darker than the regular dates you are likely used to. They are not just a tasty treat; they also have a high fiber concentration, which makes them important in healthy, rapid digestion as well as the prevention of constipation. Medjool dates prevent heart disease by functioning heavily in the removal of unhealthy fats. Research shows that dates contain a high concentration of antioxidants which retard the activities of free radicals. Medjool dates contain high concentrations of calcium, phosphorus, and magnesium, making them essential in the building and maintenance of strong bones and teeth. Medjool dates have a reasonable carbohydrate content, making them surprisingly powerful sources of energy. Isn't it refreshing to learn that they are incredibly efficient in the invigoration of existing brain cells as well as in the restoration of damaged ones? This a rare quality which makes dates essential for optimum long-term brain health and the prevention of cognitive decline as you age,

At 23 pieces per pound, you can buy a pound of Medjool dates at any local grocery store for about $10.

Parsley: Parsley is a green vegetable that is highly consumed among the natives of the Mediterranean region – one of the healthiest regions of the world, by virtue of their uniquely healthy diet. Parsley contains a healthy dose of antioxidants and anticarcinogenic biochemical, which adequately combat the oxidative effects of free radicals, and the tumor-causing effects of carcinogens. It also packs a lot of Lutein, Beta carotene, and Zeaxanthin. By this alone, Parsley makes a great sirtfood, which is significantly helpful in maintaining perfect eyesight and preventing eye defects as the body ages. Parsley's ability to help burn unhealthy fat deposits makes it key to long-term cardiac health, while its anti-bacterial properties make it important in helping the body fight infections. You can easily purchase a pound of parsley at your local grocery at under $6 per pound.

Red Endive: This is a class of veggie that contains Kaempferol, a polyphenol that promotes the burning of fats, and increased cognitive abilities. Red endives are anti-carcinogenic, boost cardiac health, improve vision, and promote optimum fetal development in pregnant women due to their high concentrations of folate. Like most sirtfoods, Red endives can be purchased at the fresh produce section of your local grocery store at $2.50 per pound.

Soybeans: Soybeans are one of the world's most prolific legumes in terms of protein content. The huge amount of pure plant protein in soybeans makes them crucial to building muscle mass and promoting the restoration and rejuvenation of body cells. Soybeans contain low fat and cholesterol levels and play significant roles in helping to reduce the accumulation of unhealthy fat deposits within the body, thereby boosting long-term cardiac health. Soybeans are also rich in Vitamin K, Folate, Copper Manganese, and Phosphorus. They have been found to possess strong anti-carcinogenic properties and have biochemicals that help alleviate the symptoms of menopause. The latter help older women transit painlessly into another phase of their lives. You can buy organic soybeans from your local grocery store at around $15 per pound.

Strawberries: Welcome the brightest and most attractive member of the sirtfoods – even though some people might argue that dark chocolate is the most attractive core sirtfood. Strawberries are sweet, juicy, and appealing, and contain huge amounts of Vitamin C, making them essential in boosting immunity and promoting the quick healing of internal and external wounds. It no accident how they promote healthy aging because of the manganese and folate antioxidants that are contained in them. Also, because of their fat-burning powers, strawberries can promote long-term cardiac well-being and control blood sugar levels. You can purchase a 2-pound pack of strawberries at your local produce store for just under $4.

Turmeric: Turmeric is one of the most respected spices in the world, and that's for a good reason. Turmeric is a natural anti-inflammatory agent, possesses natural antioxidants, and is very efficient at reducing an individual's risk of brain disease. It is also equipped with the ability to lower the risk of heart disease and cancer. The natural pain-relief agents in turmeric make it essential in the mitigation of arthritis and general muscle pains. Turmeric's natural polyphenols also have a general calming effect on the mind, helping to ward off symptoms of clinical depression. You can purchase a pound of ground turmeric at your local store for around $12.

Walnuts: Finally, we have the last but certainly

not the least on our list of core sirtfood, and what can that be if not walnuts? Walnuts are definitely one of the most medicinal species of nuts to have ever existed. They are generally regarded as great foods that can undoubtedly help a person lose weight and reduce the risk of chronic diseases. Walnuts, however, possess potent antioxidants that counteract the effects of free radicals and reduce an individual's risk of contracting Type 2 diabetes, heart disease, and cancer.

Recommended walnut brands include Great Value Chopped Walnut (24 oz.) and Fisher Chef's Natural Walnut Halves and Pieces (32 oz.), both costing about $10 and $13 respectively.

To this end, we have come to the zed of your shopping list for both phase 1 and phase 2 of the Sirtfood diet scheme. In this chapter, we have covered the health significances of the twenty core sirtfoods and why these foods have been recommended to be incorporated into your diet. As has been aforementioned, there are tons of other foods that can still be incorporated into your diet without retarding the effects of the sirtfoods. These other categories of agreeable foods will be unveiled as we forge further into the adjoining chapters.

CHAPTER SIX

BREAKFAST RECIPES

In this chapter, we would be examining the step-by-step process of creating amazing, mouth-watering sirtfood dishes that are perfect for breakfast. These foods have been carefully picked out to provide you with the energy and vigor you'd need to perform excellently all through your day while helping you to stay healthy, lose unhealthy fat, and look amazing. Let's dive right in!

SIRT MUESLI

Ingredients

- One-quarter cup of buckwheat flakes
- Two-thirds cup of buckwheat puffs
- Three tbsp. coconut flakes
- One-quarter cup Medjool dates
- One-eighth cup of chopped walnuts
- One and a half tbsp. of cocoa nibs
- Two-thirds cup of chopped strawberries
- 3/8 cup plain Greek Yoghurt

Preparation

- Simply mix all the ingredients in a clean bowl, and enjoy the fantastic goodness of this delicacy. However, only add strawberries and yogurt when you are ready to eat.

SIRTFOOD OMELET

Ingredients

- 2 oz. sliced bacon
- Three medium-sized eggs
- One and a one-quarter oz. sliced red endive
- 2 tbsp. chopped parsley
- One tsp. turmeric
- One tsp. extra virgin olive oil

Preparation

- Heat up a non-stick pan.
- Cut your bacon into thin strips.
- Cook your sliced bacon strips at high heat until they get crisp and crunchy. You do not have to add oil to the strips; the natural fat would help cook them.
- Remove the bacon strips from the pan once they're cooked, and place them on a paper towel to drain the extra fat.
- Wipe your pan clean and then pour in some oil – enough to cook the three eggs.

- Beat your eggs thoroughly and add in the turmeric, parsley, and endive.
- Chop your bacon into fine cubes and then stir the bits into the whisked eggs.
- Pour in oil into your pan and heat at medium heat.
- Pour the egg mixture in the hot oil and move the mixture around with a spatula
- Swirl the mixture carefully around the pan until the omelet is even.
- Lower the heat on your cooker and allow the omelet to firm up and even out at the edges.
- Fold your omelet in half, roll it up and serve hot.

SIRTFOOD SMOOTHIE

Ingredients

- 3/8 cup of Greek yogurt
- Six walnut halves
- 10 hulled strawberries
- 7 – 10 kale leaves
- ¾ oz. dark chocolate
- One Medjool date
- ½ tsp. ground turmeric
- One sliver of Thai chili
- 200ml of unsweetened almond milk

Preparation

- Load up all the ingredients into your blender and grind into a smooth pulp.

YOGURT, BERRIES, WALNUTS, AND DARK CHOCOLATE.

Ingredients

- One and twenty-five grams of mixed berries
- Two-thirds cup of plain Greek yogurt
- ¼ cup of walnuts
- 10g of dark chocolate (85% pure cocoa)

This recipe is extremely simple and easy to follow and features the protein-packed Greek yogurt once again.

Preparation

- Get a clean bowl and add in your berries.
- Pour the plain Greek yogurt over the berries
- Add in your walnuts and dark chocolate, and food is ready.

SEASONED SCRAMBLED EGGS

Ingredients

- One tsp. extra virgin olive oil
- 20g chopped red onions
- ½ chopped Thai chili
- 3 eggs (medium-sized)
- 50 ml of milk
- One tsp ground turmeric
- 2 tbsp. chopped parsley

This fantastic recipe allows you to relish the unbeatable taste and the amazing health benefits of scrambled eggs before you go to attack your day, fully loaded, and ready to go.

Preparation

- Place a dry, non-stick frying pan on your cooker and set to medium heat.
- Fry your chili and red onions till they get soft without being browned.
- Whisk your eggs in a clean bowl and add in the milk, parsley, and turmeric.

- Pour the mixture into the hot pan and allow to cook at medium heat
- Move the egg mixture around in the pan to scramble it and prevent burning.
- Serve once desired consistency is achieved.

ASIAN SHRIMP STIR-FRY ALONG WITH BUCKWHEAT NOODLES

Ingredients

- Two teaspoons of deveined tamari sauce
- Seventy-five grams of buckwheat noodles
- One hundred and fifty grams of shelled raw jumbo shrimp
- Two pieces of garlic cloves
- One Thai chili (it should be finely chopped)
- One teaspoon of fresh ginger (finely chopped)
- Two teaspoons of extra virgin olive oil
- Twenty grams of red onions
- Forty-five grams of celery (sliced)
- Seventy-five grams of chopped green beans
- Fifty grams of chopped kale
- Half-a-cup of chicken stock

Preparation

- Get a frying pan (non-stick) and then use a high heat setting to heat it up.
- Proceed by frying the shrimp by using a single

teaspoon of tamari sauce along with a single teaspoon of oil. Fry for four minutes.

- Have the shrimp transferred to a plate then use a clean paper towel to wipe the pan.
- In the hot water, cook the noodles for five to eight minutes, and strain.
- Proceed by frying the red onion, green beans, chili, ginger, garlic, kale and celery by using the leftover oil and tamari. Avoid including the celery leaves in that mixture. By using a medium heat setting, fry the ingredients for three-to-four minutes.
- Now include the stock to your mixture and allow it to cook till the vegs are done.
- The celery leaves, shrimp and noodles should now be added to the pan. Boil them. Once you're done, lower the heat then serve.

MISO AND SESAME GLAZED TOFU WITH GINGER AND CHILI STIR

Ingredients

- One tbsp mirin
- Twenty grams of miso paste
- One hundred and fifty grams of tofu
- Forty grams of celery
- Forty grams of red onion
- One hundred and twenty grams of zucchini
- One piece of Thai chili
- Two cloves of garlic
- One teaspoon of fresh ginger (finely chopped)
- Fifty grams of kale
- Two teaspoons of sesame seeds
- Thirty-five grams of buckwheat
- One teaspoon of ground turmeric
- Two teaspoons of extra virgin olive oil
- One teaspoon of tamari sauce

Preparation

- Heat your oven to four hundred degrees.

- Get a small roasting pan and line it with parchment paper.
- Combine the mirin and the miso.
- Slice up your tofu lengthwise, and then make each piece out into a triangular shape.
- Spread the miso mixture over the tofu and allow the tofu to get steeped in the mixture.
- Cut up your celery, red onion, and zucchini.
- Cut up the chili, garlic, and ginger.
- Allow the kale to gently cook in a steamer for five minutes.
- Transfer your tofu into the roasting pan and spread the sesame seeds over it. Allow the mixture to roast in the oven for twenty minutes.
- Rinse your buckwheat, and then sieve. Bring a pan filled with water to boil and add in the turmeric.
- Cook the buckwheat noodles and strain.
- Allow the oil to heat in a frying pan and then add the celery, onion, zucchini, chili, garlic, and ginger. Allow the entire mix to fry on high heat for two minutes. Reduce the heat to medium for four minutes until the vegetables are cooked.

- Add a tablespoon of water if the vegetables get stuck to the pan. Spread in the kale and tamari and allow the mixture to cook for another minute.
- Serve the cooked tofu with the greens and the buckwheat.

TURKEY ESCALOPE ALONG WITH SAGE, SPICED CAULIFLOWER, PARSLEY & CAPERS

Ingredients

- One hundred and fifty grams of chopped cauliflower
- Two garlic cloves
- Forty grams of red onions
- Two garlic cloves
- One Thai chili
- One teaspoon of chopped fresh ginger
- Two tablespoons of extra virgin olive oil
- Two teaspoons ground turmeric
- Thirty grams of sun-dried tomatoes
- Ten grams of fresh parsley
- One hundred and fifty grams of turkey steak
- One teaspoon of dried sage juice
- One-quarter lemon
- One tablespoon of capers

Preparation

- Put the raw cauliflower into your food processor.
- Chop up the cauliflower until a fine consistency is achieved.
- Fry the ginger, garlic, chili and red onions and ginger in the extra virgin olive oil until they are all reasonably soft.
- Put in your turmeric and cauliflower at this point, and allow the entire mixture to cook for one minute.
- Bring the mixture down form your cooker, then add the tomatoes and half of your parsley.
- Cover your turkey escalope with oil and sage and fry for six minutes, making sure to turn carefully to prevent burning.
- At this point, proceed by pouring in the lemon juice, parsley, capers, and one tablespoon of water to the pan to create your sauce.

BUCKWHEAT PANCAKES, MUSHROOMS, RED ONIONS, AND KALE SALAD

Ingredients

- One buckwheat pancake
- 50g button mushrooms
- Fifteen grams of chicken
- 200g Kale
- 20g red onions
- Extra Virgin Olive Oil

Preparation

- Clean and cut the button mushrooms.
- Clean and cut the kale into thin strips and the red onions into rings. Combine the green cabbage and onion in a bowl, season with a drizzle of olive oil, and possibly a little lemon.
- Cut the chicken into pieces. In a pan, arrange a drizzle of olive oil and add the chicken pieces.
- Add the mushrooms and brown them.
- Place everything in the buckwheat pancake,

and close the pancake.

- On a plate, arrange the green cabbage / red onion salad, then place the hot buckwheat pancake next to it. Enjoy your meal!

NAAN BREAD WITH BAKED TOFU AND CAULIFLOWER

Ingredients

- 50 g firm plain tofu
- 50 g cauliflower
- ½ clove garlic
- ½ small onion
- 50ml of water
- 50ml coconut milk
- ½ tablespoon of tomato puree
- ½ teaspoon powdered Indian broth
- ½ tablespoon coconut oil
- ½ teaspoon curry powder
- ½ teaspoon cumin
- ½ tablespoon potato starch

Naan bread:

- 75g wheat flour
- One plain yogurt
- Two pinches of sugar
- 5g baker's yeast or 8 g dehydrated yeast

- 5g salt
- Two tablespoons extra virgin olive oil
- 5 cl lukewarm water
- One teaspoon caraway seeds

Preparation

- Peel and mince the garlic and the onions.
- In a casserole dish, sauté everything in coconut oil with the curry and cumin until lightly colored.
- Add the coconut milk, the tomato puree, and 50 ml of water and the Indian broth. Mix well then bring to a dainty simmer.
- Add the tofu pieces and the cauliflower.
- Cook gently without the lid on for about 20 min until the cauliflower is slightly tender.
- Dilute the starch with a little cooking juice, then pour back into the casserole dish and continue cooking for 5 min.
- Serve with basmati rice and naan bread.

Naan Bread

- Put the flour in your food processor.
- Add the crumbled yeast, olive oil, sugar, yogurt, caraway seeds, and mix well.
- Proceed by adding the water and continue

mixing with the whisk until the dough is soft and comes off the sides of your bowl.

- Now place the ball of dough in a small bowl then cover, and allow to stand for thirty minutes.
- Heat up an empty pan, and cook the naan bread on each side for four minutes to remove moisture.
- Enjoy your mouth-watering delicacy.

CHAPTER SEVEN

SUGGESTED LUNCH RECIPES

In this chapter, we would be reviewing in detail the ingredients and steps needed to prepare some of the most delicious and healthy sirtfoods suitable for lunch.

SALMON FILLET, ENDIVE, ARUGULA AND CELERY

Ingredients

- 200g fresh salmon fillet
- 200g arugula
- Three red endives
- One large pink grapefruit
- Two slices of smoked salmon
- One small shallot
- One lemon
- Grated Parmesan cheese
- Extra virgin olive oil
- One teaspoon balsamic vinegar
- Salt and pepper to taste

Preparation

- Cut the lemon in half to gently extract the liquid juice inside it.
- Peel the grapefruit over a bowl to collect the juice. Detach the quarters and cut them into pieces.

- Peel and chop the shallot.
- Remove the skin and bones from the fresh salmon fillet, then dice into small pieces
- Place the whole mixture in a salad bowl, sprinkle with the lime and grapefruit juice, mix and let stand aside.
- Cut the bottoms of the endives, remove the damaged leaves, and chop the main parts into thin strips.
- Wash and wring the arugula.
- Carefully cut the smoked salmon slices into light strips.
- Drain the marinated salmon fillet well, and keep two teaspoons of the marinade.
- Emulsify the marinade with olive oil and balsamic vinegar in a bowl, then salt and pepper as desired.
- In a salad bowl, mix the diced salmon fillet, the smoked salmon strips, the pieces of grapefruit, the arugula, the minced endives, and the olive oil sauce. Turn to mix and sprinkle lightly with grated Parmesan cheese.
- Serve this salad immediately and serve with slices of toast. Do not hesitate to double the proportions if you want to enjoy it as a main dish.

TUSCAN BEAN STEW

Ingredients

- Two teaspoons extra virgin olive oil
- 6 oz. cooked chicken sausages cut lengthwise in half and sliced
- 10 oz. fresh mushrooms
- One small raw red onion
- Two thinly sliced garlic cloves
- 29 oz. canned, diced tomatoes
- Sixteen oz. canned beans
- One medium uncooked zucchini
- One tbsp. rosemary
- ¼ tsp salt
- 2 oz. arugula
- ¼ cups Grated Parmesan Cheese

Preparation

- By using a Dutch oven, set the heat level to medium-high.
- Add the sausages and cook, often stirring, until

lightly browned, about three minutes.

- Using a cooking spoon, transfer to a small bowl or plate.
- Add the mushrooms and onion to the pot and cook, often stirring, until the vegetables are tender, usually for about three minutes.
- Now add the garlic and cook, constantly stirring for about 30 seconds.
- Add the sausages to the tomatoes, beans, zucchini, rosemary, and salt and allow to boil.
- Lower the heat and simmer, till the mushrooms becomes soft, usually after about 2 minutes.
- Remove from heat and stir in the arugula until it is softened.
- Pour the stew into four bowls and garnish evenly with Parmesan.

STRAWBERRY BUCKWHEAT SALAD

Ingredients

Tamari dressing:

- One-quarter cup of olive oil
- Two tablespoons of vinegar
- One tablespoon of reduced salt tamari sauce
- One tablespoon of old-fashioned mustard

Salad:

- One cup buckwheat, rinsed and drained
- 6 cups mixed lettuce
- 2 cups strawberries, hulled and sliced
- A half fennel bulb cut into thin slices
- One-third cup of red onion, cut into thin strips
- Six cooked bacon slices, chopped
- One-third cup of roasted sunflower seeds
- Salt and pepper

Preparation

Tamari vinaigrette:

- In a small jar, put the olive oil, rice vinegar,

tamari sauce, and old-fashioned mustard. Add in some pepper.

- Close the lid and shake vigorously.

Salad preparation

- Now place the buckwheat in a medium-sized bowl and cover with at least 2 inches (5 cm) of water. Cover the bowl and let soak in the refrigerator overnight. Drain buckwheat, rinse with cold water, and drain again.
- In a large bowl, put the lettuce, strawberries, fennel, onion, bacon, sunflower seeds, and reserved buckwheat. Add in your dressing and mix well.

SAUTÉED POTATOES IN CHICKEN BROTH

Ingredients

- Six medium-sized potatoes
- One onion
- Chicken broth
- 100ml of water
- One tbsp extra virgin olive oil
- Salt to taste

Preparation

- First peel the potatoes then slice it across into pieces.
- Proceed by peeling the onions and chop into small pieces.
- Fry minced onion pieces in oil for five minutes. Add in the potatoes and cook for another ten minutes while stirring gently.
- Dilute the chicken broth with water and add to the cooker, and cook for five minutes.
- Add salt to taste and serve.

BAKED POTATOES AND CHILI CON CARNE

Ingredients

- 8Big potatoes
- 600g Knife ground beef
- 35cl Beef broth
- 500g Crushed tomatoes
- 500g Canned kidney beans
- 1 tbsp. Tomato puree
- 2 Big onions
- One bunch of chives
- Two garlic cloves
- Half teaspoon Chili powder
- One tbsp. Cumin
- One tbsp. dried oregano
- 2 tbsp. Extra Virgin Olive Oil
- 250g Farm fresh cream
- Salt and pepper to taste

Preparation

- Peel and chop the onions and garlic.

- Heat the broth in a saucepan.
- Heat the oil available in the frying pan to fry the onions and garlic for five minutes while mixing.
- Add the meat and allow to cook for five minutes over high heat. Add salt and pepper.
- Pour the tomatoes and the tomato puree, then the broth.
- Add the cumin, oregano, and chili, and then mix. Cover and simmer 45 minutes.
- Add the beans, cover, and continue cooking over low heat, 20 min.
- Preheat the oven to 180 ° C
- Wash the potatoes. Once done, wrap them together in aluminum foil and bake for 30 to 35 minutes.
- Remove the paper, cut the potatoes in half and scoop it out slightly to garnish with chili.
- Top each potato with a spoonful of cream
- Serve hot.

CHICKEN IN PEPPER SAUCE

Ingredients

- One jar of 340 ml roasted peppers
- One cup (250 mL) canned coconut milk
- Fifteen ml red wine vinegar
- Two cloves of garlic
- One tsp. paprika
- One tsp. dried oregano
- One tsp. salt
- One-quarter cup of chopped fresh parsley, chopped
- One tbsp extra virgin olive oil
- Four boneless skinless chicken breasts or thighs
- Salt and pepper
- One minced onion
- One red bell pepper (minced)
- One-quarter cup of chopped fresh parsley, for garnish

Preparation

- In a blender, mix all the ingredients for the sauce (everything above except chicken, olive oil, onions, salt, and pepper) until you get a mixture of smooth consistency.
- Place a rack at the center of your oven and preheat to 400 ° F.
- In your large non-stick skillet (you can use a cast iron), heat the olive oil over high heat and fry the chicken breasts. Generously season with salt and pepper. Give it time by allowing all the sides of the chicken to fry for at least three minutes and then set aside on a plate.
- Lower the heat level back to medium then add the onions, and allow to heat for six minutes over medium heat, stirring often.
- Add the red pepper and cook for another minute only.
- Return the chicken to the pan and sprinkle with the roasted pepper sauce.
- Bake the dish for fifteen minutes. Before serving, remove from the oven and grace it by adding some parsley. Serve with pasta in olive oil and chives or white rice.

WALDORF SALAD

Ingredients

- One hundred and twenty-five grams of mayonnaise
- Two tablespoons white vinegar
- One apple, peeled and cut into pieces
- One celery stalk, diced
- One hundred and twenty-five grams of grapes
- One hundred and twenty-five grams of chopped walnuts
- Salt and pepper to taste

Preparation

- In a large bowl, whisk the mayonnaise and vincgar.
- Add the apple, celery, raisins, and walnuts.
- Sprinkle in salt and pepper. Mix everything and serve fresh.

WHOLE WHEAT PITA

Ingredients

- 250g of whole wheat flour
- 2 tbsp extra virgin olive oil
- 5g salt
- 10g dry baker's yeast
- One hundred and fifty-ml hot water

Preparation

- Add the whole flour and the salt in a bowl and stir. Then add the rest of the ingredients: oil, yeast, and water. Stir thoroughly to mix.
- Mix all the ingredients well until the pita bread dough is formed. Knead the dough for a few minutes on the table. If the dough seem to be too dry, you can add a little more water.
- Once kneaded, make the dough into a ball and put it in a bowl. Have it covered and let it be there for two hours.
- Take out the whole pita bread dough and knead again. Work the dough into balls of about 80g each. Use a roller to make the dough well-

rounded. Make the pieces of bread ten-to-twelve cm wide and One cm thick.

- Put the pitas on a tray. Preheat the oven to 200 ° C, slot in the tray, and let the pieces of bread bake for ten minutes, depending on the oven.
- Finally, take out the pieces of bread, let them cool a little and serve!

SCRAMBLED TOFU WITH MUSHROOMS (VEGAN)

Ingredients

- One hundred and twenty-five grams of plain firm tofu
- 100g silky tofu
- One tbsp. fresh cream
- One tbsp. sesame puree
- One tsp. Mustard
- ½ tsp. ground turmeric
- Four sprigs of fresh chives
- Half onion (optional)
- One garlic clove (optional)
- 50g mushrooms
- 2 tbsp. Extra Virgin Olive Oil
- One tbsp. Tamari soy sauce (gluten-free, organic soy sauce)
- Salt and pepper to taste

Preparation

- In a bowl, crush the firm tofu, add in the silky

tofu, cream, tahini, mustard, turmeric, and chopped chives.

- Mix thoroughly, and add salt and pepper to taste.
- Peel and chop the onion and the garlic.
- Rinse the mushrooms under a stream of water. Cut off the ends of the stalks and cut the mushrooms into strips. Gently fry the mushrooms, onions, and garlic over medium-high heat in a pan with a little olive oil.
- Once the mushrooms, onions, and garlic are very tender and slightly brown in color, add the mixture to the tofu and cook over medium heat for about 5 minutes. Stir the mixture continuously with a spatula.
- Serve hot, and enjoy.

PASTA WITH SMOKED SALMON AND ARUGULA

Ingredients

- 250g Spaghetti
- One hundred and fifty grams of Smoked salmon
- One bunch of arugula
- 2 tbsp. Extra virgin olive oil
- One finely chopped onion
- Salt and pepper to taste

Preparation

- Cook the pasta in boiling water for ten minutes. Add salt to taste.
- Slice the smoked salmon into strips. Rinse and wring the arugula.
- Heat One tablespoonful of extra virgin olive oil in a frying pan and chop the onion. Add in the drained spaghetti, the salmon strips, and the arugula. Mix well and cook for 2 min.
- Sprinkle in the rest of the olive oil, salt, and

pepper.

- Mix and serve hot.

CHAPTER EIGHT

SUGGESTED DINNER RECIPES

In this chapter, we would be reviewing ten amazing sirtfood recipes that can ideally be made for dinner.

FUSILLI SALAD WITH BUCKWHEAT, PESTO, TOMATOES, AND PINE NUTS

Ingredients

- 200g buckwheat fusilli
- Sixteen cherry tomatoes
- 80g dried tomatoes
- 40g pine nuts

- Salt and pepper
- 4 tbsp. basil pesto

Basil Pesto:

- One bunch of basil
- 2 tbsp. olive oil
- 50g parmesan
- 60g pine nuts
- One clove of garlic all mixed

Preparation

- Cook the pasta for ten minutes, add salt to taste. Drain and let it cool.
- Cut the cherry tomatoes in half, chop the dried tomatoes into thin strips and lightly toast the pine nuts in a pan for one minute.
- In a large bowl, gently mix the pasta and pesto. Add the dried tomatoes, half of the chopped basil and the pine nuts. Carefully stir the entire mixture and add seasoning to taste.
- Arrange the cherry tomatoes and the rest of the chopped basil on the salad.

TOFU AND MUSHROOM SOUP

Ingredients

- 500ml vegetable broth (or 500 ml of water and One tbsp. dehydrated vegetable broth)
- 375ml Soy beverage
- 250g button mushrooms ready to use
- 240g herb tofu
- 4 tbsp. tapioca
- One medium onion
- One tbsp. canola oil
- One tbsp. parsley
- Pepper to taste

Preparation

- Rinse the mushrooms thoroughly and cut them into pieces.
- Peel the onion and dice it.
- Heat the oil over medium heat in a saucepan. Sauté the onion in the oil for one minute, and then add the mushrooms and cook for five minutes, stirring occasionally.

- While the mushrooms and onion cook cut the diced tofu, and wash and chop your parsley.
- Add the vegetable broth and soy beverage to the mixture cooking.
- Add the tapioca into the mixture, then add the tofu. Continue cooking over low heat for about seven minutes.
- Sprinkle with chopped parsley and serve.

SALMON SALAD AND FRESH MINT

Ingredients

- Salad leaves
- 200 g of fresh salmon
- Six mint leaves
- Three tablespoons of white cheese
- Two limes
- Salad dressing
- One large cucumber

Preparation

- Peel the cucumber and remove the seeds. Cut the cucumber into thin rings and put it in a colander.
- Steam your salmon for 8 minutes. Mash the salmon in a bowl and mix in the cottage cheese with the lemon, salt, and pepper
- Add the chopped mint, mix well, and refrigerate.
- Place the salad in strips on a plate and add in the cucumber salmon and enjoy!

GRANOLA WITH HAZELNUTS AND CHOCOLATE CHIPS

Ingredients

- Four small oatmeal packs
- 2 tbsp. coconut oil
- Two whole hazelnut packs
- One 200 bar of dark chocolate
- 4 tbsp maple syrup

Preparation

- Preheat your oven to 150°C
- Cut your hazelnuts and chocolate bar into small pieces.
- In a medium-sized bowl, mix the oats, coconut oil, hazelnut chips, and the maple syrup to give a paste.
- Spread the paste over a sheet of baking paper. Keep the thickness at half a centimeter at most.
- Bake halfway and cook for about thirty minutes until the mixture is slightly brown.
- Take the baking sheet out of the oven and,

using a zester or a cheese grater, grind the whole four squares of chocolate you have kept whole. Make it right out of the oven when the dough is still hot.

- Allow to cool and mix your granola with the chocolate chips.

CHICKEN TAGINE WITH SQUASH AND MEDJOOL DATES

Ingredients

- One large chicken cut into eight pieces
- 4 tbsp. extra virgin olive oil
- 2 tbsp flaked almonds
- Two chopped onions
- One.5 tsp ground cumin
- One tsp coriander seeds
- One tbsp. ground cinnamon
- Two garlic cloves (chopped)
- Two slices of fresh ginger
- One sachet of saffron
- Salt and pepper to taste
- 500 ml chicken broth
- 750g peeled squash
- Six large pitted dates cut in half
- One bunch of fresh coriander
- Orange zest

Preparation

- Leniently toast the almonds in your frying pan and set aside.
- Proceed by heating a little fraction of oil in a Dutch oven and fry the onions for about five-to-six minutes, continue stirring until they are slightly brown.
- Add in the cumin, previously crushed coriander seeds, cinnamon, and garlic. Now cook for roughly two minutes then add the chicken, ginger and saffron, salt, and pepper.
- Cover the entire mixture with chicken broth and bake in a covered oven for One hour.
- Add the squash, dates, and orange zest. Continue cooking for about 20-25 minutes.
- Remove the ginger and serve on a bed of couscous. Add in the cooking broth and garnish with chopped fresh coriander and toasted almonds.

SHRIMP AND ARRABBIATA SAUCE

Ingredients

- One onion, chopped
- One tsp crushed hot pepper flakes
- 5 tbsp. Extra Virgin Olive Oil
- Two garlic cloves, chopped
- 60 ml white wine
- 28 oz. crushed Italian tomatoes
- 375g pasta
- 454g large raw shrimp (peeled)
- 2 tbsp Chopped parsley
- One cup grated Parmesan Cheese
- Salt and pepper

Preparation

- Get a saucepan then add the three tablespoons of oil, sauté the onion and the pepper in the oil then heat. You should also add some pepper and salt to taste.
- Add the garlic and continue cooking for One minute. Deglaze with white wine.

- Add the tomatoes and continue cooking for about ten minutes.
- Boil your pasta. Add in a little salt and oil. Drain and serve.
- In a large skillet heated over high heat, heat the shrimp in hot oil. Add salt and pepper to taste.
- Add the sauce and allow the mixture to boil.
- Add the pasta and parsley and season to taste.
- Serve warm. You can also shower it with Parmesan cheese if desired.

TURMERIC SALMON AND COCONUT MILK

Ingredients

- Two skinless salmon steaks
- One onion
- One garlic clove
- One tsp. turmeric
- 10 cl coconut milk
- 10 cl of fish stock
- 4 tbsp. Extra Virgin Olive oil
- Salt and pepper to taste

Preparation

- Peel and chop the onion and garlic. Fry on low heat for 3 minutes in a saucepan with two tablespoons of olive oil.
- Add the turmeric, cook for 30 seconds, and then pour the coconut milk and the fish stock.
- Add in pepper and salt to taste and cook over very low heat for 10 minutes.
- Cook the salmon steaks over high heat in a pan

with two tablespoons of olive oil. Cook each side for One to 2 minutes.

- Serve the fish with the sauce.

CORONATION CHICKEN SALAD WITH CHEESE

Ingredients

- 200g chicken cutlet
- One hundred and seventy-five grams of spelled flour
- 75g cottage cheese
- 50g ground almonds
- Three eggs
- One onion
- Half tsp. baking powder
- 2 tbsp. Extra Virgin Olive Oil
- 10 cl whole milk
- One tbsp. pepper
- One tsp. nutmeg

Preparation

- Warm by using the extra virgin olive oil in a non-stick pan, add the minced onions and the diced chicken and allow the mixture to fry until slightly brown.

- Melt the cheese in a bowl, add the eggs, flour, yeast, oil, and warm milk.
- Add the mixture to the chicken. Sprinkle in the pepper, nutmeg, and finally, the powdered almonds.
- Mix well, then pour the dough into a mold and bake for about 40 minutes in an oven preheated to One80 ° C.
- Serve warm with a salad.

BAKED POTATOES AND CHICKPEA STEW

Ingredients

- 4-6 baking potatoes
- One tbsp. canola oil
- One tbsp. cumin seeds
- One red onion (finely chopped)
- Five garlic cloves (minced)
- One tbsp. ground coriander seeds
- One can of chickpeas (drained)
- One cup of water
- One red potato (diced)
- 2 tsp. chopped fresh cilantro
- Half tsp. salt
- Half tsp. coarsely ground pepper
- One tomato (diced)

Preparation

- Preheat your oven to 200°C, and add in your baking potatoes for an hour.
- By using a medium-high heat settings for the

saucepan, heat the oil in it to fry the cumin seeds for 10 seconds till they are slightly brown, then add the onion and garlic and stir till they are slightly brown too. Finally, add the coriander and stir for another thirty seconds.

- Add the chickpeas, water, potato, and one tsp. of fresh cilantro. Add in salt and pepper to taste.
- Lower the heat and boil the entire mixture. Cover then simmer for fifteen minutes till the potato is soft.
- Proceed by adding the diced tomatoes then increase the heat slightly. Allow cooking for One-to-two minutes.
- Garnish with the leftover fresh cilantro and serve with the baked potatoes.

CHICKEN SALAD WITH SESAME SEEDS

Ingredients

- Two chicken strips
- Mixed salad (Californian style)
- One onion (finely chopped)
- One tbsp. sesame seeds
- One tsp. Almonds
- One tbsp. Dijon's mustard
- 2 tbsp. Extra Virgin Olive oil
- One tbsp. Balsamic vinegar
- One Lemon
- Bacon (to taste)

Preparation

- Warm by using the extra virgin olive oil in a non-stick pan over high heat.
- Fry the chicken breasts in the pan with a little mustard to add flavor.
- Prepare the vinaigrette with oil, balsamic vinegar, finely chopped onions, and a little

mustard. Stir the mixture thoroughly and leave to marinate.

- Wash and cut the salad leaves, and then mix the salad and the vinaigrette.
- Cut the chicken strips into thin slices.
- Peel the bacon and place everything on the salad.
- Sprinkle in the almonds and sesame seeds. Add fresh lemon zest to taste.

CHAPTER NINE

SIRTFOOD SNACKS AND DESSERTS

It is imminent that at some points during your day, you would feel a pang hunger and have the urge to grab a snack. If you are the kind of person that used to eat a lot of junk foods before, the healthy snacks and desserts classified as sirtfood bites can help you to prevent relapsing into eating unhealthy foods, as they are portable, fill you up temporarily and are delectably tasty. In this chapter, we would be reviewing ten sirtfood snacks and desserts.

GREEN TEA

Ingredients

- One tbsp. green tea powder
- One cup of water

Preparation

- Simply dissolve the green tea powder in the glass of water and enjoy it.

RED GRAPES

Ingredients

- 5 – 10 pieces of red grapes

Preparation

- Simply rinse the grapes under running water and enjoy.

APPLES

Ingredients

- 2 -3 Apples

Preparation

- Simply rinse your Apples under running water and enjoy

DARK CHOCOLATE

Ingredients

- One bar of 85% dark cocoa chocolate

Preparation

- Remove the dark chocolate from its wrapping and slowly savor with water or green tea.

COCOA

Ingredients

- Two tsp. of pure cocoa powder
- One cup of water
- 30ml milk
- One tsp. sugar

Preparation

- Pour in the cocoa, milk, and sugar into the glass.
- In your kettle, warm the water inside it, or get some water out of your refrigerator.
- Mix the water and the mixture in the cup, and enjoy it.

OLIVES

Ingredients

- Six large black or green olives

Preparation

- Simply rinse the olives under running water, and serve at room temperature.

BLACKBERRIES

Ingredients

- Ten-to-fifteen blackberries

Preparation

- For optimum satisfaction, keep your blackberries refrigerated for four to five hours, and enjoy chilled.

POMEGRANATE SEEDS

Ingredients

- 50g pomegranate seeds

Preparation

- Unleash the goodness of this healthy sirtfood snack by simply popping half of a pack in your mouth when you feel hungry in the middle of the day, or after a meal.

BLUEBERRIES

Ingredients

- 25 pieces of blueberries

Preparation

- Simply rinse your berries under running water, or retrieve from your refrigerator after four to five hours, and enjoy.

STRAWBERRIES

Ingredients

- 50g of strawberries

Preparation

- Keep the strawberries refrigerated for a few hours, and enjoy as a fruity snack or dessert.

CHAPTER TEN

21-DAYS MEAL PLAN

Experts in psychology have proven repeatedly over the years that it takes 21 days for the average human being to build a habit, and 90 days for that habit to become fully incorporated into his lifestyle. Building a habit can be challenging if you do not have a solid game plan, and that is our ambition for this chapter. In this chapter, we would build a 21-days sirtfood timetable that would help you get through Phases One and Two of the Sirtfood diet. Let's get moving!

PHASE ONE

DAY 1:

Breakfast: Sirtfood Green Juice

Lunch: Sirt Muesli

Dinner: Sirtfood Green Juice

DAY 2:

Breakfast: Sirtfood Green Juice

Lunch: Spicy scrambled eggs

Dinner: Sirtfood Green Juice

DAY 3:

Breakfast: Sirtfood Green Juice

Lunch: Buckwheat Pasta Salad

Dinner: Sirtfood Green Juice

DAY 4:

Breakfast: Mushroom and Tofu Scramble

Lunch: Sirtfood smoothie

Dinner: Sirtfood Green Juice

DAY 5:

Breakfast: Sirt Tuna Salad

Lunch: Pasta with Smoked Salmon and Arugula

Dinner: Sirtfood Green Juice

DAY 6:

Breakfast: Sirtfood Omelet

Lunch: Salmon Fillet, Endive, Arugula, and Celery

Dinner: Sirtfood Green Juice

DAY 7:

Breakfast: Yoghurt, Berries, Dark Chocolate & Walnuts

Lunch: Tuscan Bean Stew

Dinner: Sirtfood Green Juice

PHASE TWO

DAY 8:

Breakfast: Seasoned Scrambled Eggs

Lunch: Strawberry Buckwheat Salad

Dinner: Fusilli Salad with Buckwheat, Tomatoes, Pesto and Pine nuts

DAY 9:

Breakfast: The Common Asian Shrimp Stir-Fry along with Buckwheat Noodles

Lunch: Sautéed Potatoes in Chicken Broth

Dinner: Tofu and Mushroom Soup

DAY 10:

Breakfast: The miso & Sesame Glazed Tofu along with Ginger & Chili Stir

Lunch: Baked Potatoes and Chili Con Carne

Dinner: Salmon Salad and Fresh Mint

DAY 11:

Breakfast: Sage along with Turkey Escalope, Spiced Cauliflower, Parsley and Capers

Lunch: Chicken in Pepper Sauce

Dinner: Granola with Hazelnuts and Chocolate Chips

DAY 12:

Breakfast: Buckwheat Pancakes, Mushrooms, Red Onions & Kale Salad

Lunch: Waldorf Salad

Dinner: Chicken Tagine with Squash and Medjool Dates

DAY 13:

Breakfast: Naan Bread with Baked Tofu and

Cauliflower

Lunch: Whole Wheat Pita

Dinner: Shrimp and Arrabbiata Sauce

DAY 14:

Breakfast: Sirt Muesli

Lunch: Scrambled Tofu with Mushrooms

Dinner: Turmeric Salmon and Coconut Milk

DAY 15:

Breakfast: Sirtfood Omelet

Lunch: Pasta with Smoked Salmon and Arugula

Dinner: Coronation Chicken Salad with Cheese

DAY 16:

Breakfast: Sirtfood smoothie

Lunch: Salmon Fillet, Arugula, Endive, and Celery

Dinner: Baked Potatoes and Chickpea Stew

DAY 17:

Breakfast: Yogurt, Berries, Dark Chocolate & Walnuts

Lunch: Tuscan Bean Stew

Dinner: Chicken Salad with Sesame Seeds

DAY 18:

Breakfast: Seasoned Scrambled Eggs

Lunch: Strawberry Buckwheat Salad

Dinner: Tofu and Mushroom Soup

DAY 19:

Breakfast: Asian Shrimp Stir-Fry with Buckwheat Noodles

Lunch: Sautéed Potatoes in Chicken Broth

Dinner: Salmon Salad and Fresh Mint

DAY 20:

Breakfast: Miso and Sesame Glazed Tofu with Ginger and Chili Stir

Lunch: Baked Potatoes and Chili Con Carne

Dinner: Granola with Hazelnuts and Chocolate Chips

DAY 21:

Breakfast: Turkey Escalope along with Sage, Spiced Cauliflower, Parsley & Capers

Lunch: Chicken in Pepper Sauce

Dinner: Chicken Tagine with Squash and Medjool Dates

CHAPTER ELEVEN

TROUBLESHOOTING AND FREQUENTLY ASKED QUESTIONS

Life is rarely ever a bed of roses, and most times, before significant victories are recorded, intense sacrifices need to be made. The sirtfood diet may seem simple and easily practicable on paper; however, when it comes to the actual execution, a couple of common problems seems to rear their heads. In this chapter, we would be examining some of the common problems that most individuals face during the course of the diet and how these challenges can be handled in the long run. We would also be answering some of the most frequently asked questions about the sirtfood diet.

Troubleshooting

1. The Problem of Cravings

In today's 'sweet' modern world, a lot of people are severely hooked on junk food and sugary snacks, and this addiction poses one of the strongest problems against progress in the sirtfood diet. Weight loss and heavy consumption of processed sugar just don't go together. As has been reiterated in the past chapters, when you consume a lot of processed sugar, your blood sugar levels rise accordingly, leading to a corresponding rise in your insulin levels. Elevated insulin levels lead to accumulated fat deposits. If you really desire the trim body, fitness, agility, and mental alertness that comes with staying steadfast through the sirtfood diet, then you must break your bad habit of compulsively consuming processed sugar.

One proven way to help you break your unhealthy addiction to sugar is to keep busy. Irrespective of where you're; home or school, be sure to keep yourself gainfully occupied doing something. Planning out your day right from the start can help to prevent situations where you end up unnecessarily idle and start considering getting a cake or an ice cream. Stay busy, productive, and focus, and your cravings will take a nosedive.

Drinking your sirtfood juice constantly throughout the first phase of the sirtfood diet and afterward would also help you keep your cravings at bay. The sirtfood green juice is packed with a variety of leafy greens that supply your body with essential nutrients and vitamins that keep you invigorated. The sirtfood juice does not only help you stay healthy; it provides you with an alternative you can turn to when the cravings come calling. To help you resist the urge to indulge in your sugary treats, you can also take advantage of the sirtfood bites described earlier in this book. Packing a box of blueberries or a bar of dark chocolate in your backpack of handbag can help provide you with something healthy to munch on as you work to prevent your cravings from overwhelming you.

Your mind will be your most powerful asset as you embark on the sirtfood diet. You need to imbibe self-discipline and constantly remind yourself of why you started this journey in the first place. Never forget that success in life is all about sacrifices, and the sacrifice you would have to make for long-term well-being is letting go of the sweet but deadly things holding you back. The realization that the desperate cravings would die down soon is also one that you need to keep at the back of your mind as you go through every single day of your sirtfood diet.

Finally, to help you win this war against your cravings, try as much as possible to distance yourself from your triggers. If you have a stash of cupcakes, muffins, or ice cream in your refrigerator, it may be time to give those foods out. Inform your friends about your new diet, so theta they can encourage you when your resolve goes weak, and so that they can control their consumption of sugary treats around you. As much as possible, it is advisable for you to avoid places like pastry shops and ice cream shacks in the early days of your diet so that you do not falter.

2. The Problem of Hunger

Hunger is another extremely common obstacle to success in the sirtfood diet, especially in phase One, where stringent calorie restrictions exist. To help you deal with the problem of hunger, try to deal with less physically exerting activities as your body gets used to surviving on lower calories. Don't push your body to the limits at this time. Keep your exercise light and rest as much as possible. Keeping your sirtfood juice handy also helps you to refuel from time to time, and helps to curb the hunger and exhaustion. Closely related to the problem of hunger during the first few days of the diet is the issue of fatigue and exhaustion.

When hunger comes around, tiredness and inactivity almost automatically follow. So to help you stay strong in your first few days of this diet, rest as much as possible, avoid extreme physical exertion, and of course, don't forget to drink your sirtfood juice.

3. The Problem of Relapsing

A lot of people go into diets with one single aim: Not to relapse. It is good to keep it in mind that you have to inculcate the self-discipline needed to pull off the rigorous sirtfood diet. However, your main aim should be to last as long as possible and eventually integrate the sirtfood diet into your lifestyle. People make mistakes and slip once or twice sometimes. Forgive yourself, pick yourself back up, and keep moving. Note that this is not a license for you to go ahead and start sneaking ice cream into your mouth on the third day of your diet. This is simply to let you realize that if you make a mistake, that doesn't mean your diet is over. Pick yourself back up, remove as much of the negative triggers as possible from your environment, and be determined to achieve your long-term health goals.

4. Being Unsure of What to Eat

The sirtfood diet contains a wonderfully wide

variety of healthy foods. We understand that picking out exactly what to eat on one particular day might be quite challenging since you might be new to most of the foods on the list. This is why we have designed the 2One-day meal plan in the previous chapter for you to refer to. If you have a designed meal plan available, you don't need to stress yourself out trying to decide what to eat. Simply consult your guide and get cooking.

5. **Being Too Busy to Cook**

Factualism has it clear that we live in a very fast-paced world where a lot of people have to battle with insane deadlines and mind-numbing workloads. We understand that finding the time to cook three times a day under these conditions may be difficult. So, we recommend that you cook some of your meals in advance, keep them in your refrigerator, and simply get microwave them if necessary before eating. For those early mornings when you need to quickly dash out, you can choose some of the simpler recipes such as the Sirt Muesli, the Sirtfood Smoothie, the Sirtfood Omelet, the spicy scrambled eggs, and other simpler options that require minimal preparation time and efforts. Success in any endeavor in the modern world is all about flexibility, and the sirtfood diet provides you with a lot of that.

6. The Temptation to Eat Out

It is a comprehensible fact that you would miss your old diners and restaurants as you begin to settle into your sirtfood diet routine. Perhaps, you even used to go out with your friends to have dinner at a specific restaurant. Once your first two phases are over, you can eat out, but ensure to eat plant-rich dishes, avoid bread and fried foods, eat slowly, and be sure to stop when you are full. Once again, having a reliable support system comes in handy in this situation. Let your friends understand that you are going through a particularly tasking diet, and you would like them to help you stay steadfast in your goals.

7. The Problem of Over-eating

As humans, our appetites differ from one person to another. However, eating too much wouldn't do you too much good in the long run. It is not compulsory for you to finish your entire plate of food. Once you are 80% full, let the remaining food go. Don't allow guilt to overwhelm you and force you back down a road of obesity and unhealthiness. Also, watch your pace of eating. If you're always in haste when eating, you are likely to over-eat. So, eat slowly instead, and note your level of satiety. Once you feel full and energized, stop. This will help you curb the problem of eating too much and overloading your body with calories.

8. Alcohol Addiction

If you are excessively addicted to alcohol, then successfully integrating the sirtfood diet into your lifestyle and reaping its amazing benefits may be extremely challenging. For a start, try to focus your time and energy on other productive activities. When the urge to drink hits, find something else – something productive and engaging – to do. Being associated to support group such as the Alcoholics Anonymous groups may also help you gradually let go of this bad habit. Keeping your friends in the loop about your decision to quit drinking will also go a long way in helping to keep your cravings for alcohol in check. Avoid pubs and bars as much as possible, and if the problem persists, then you might need to take to a medical expert about what to do to eradicate your addiction to alcohol.

Other Frequently Asked Questions

1. Should I exercise while on the Sirtfood diet?

Yes, of course! Light workouts increase the

efficiency of the sirtfood diet and help you progress faster on your journey to losing weight, achieving enhanced mental clarity, and reducing the risk of long-term chronic diseases. So, keep your workouts simple, limit physical exertion, but try as much as possible to exercise every single day.

2. Can the Sirtfood Diet rectify extreme obesity?

A lot of people believe that diets only work for overweight people, and full-blown obesity can only be corrected by surgical procedures. The decision of whether you need surgery to remove the excess fat deposits would depend on your doctor. However, if your cardiac health is not in immediate danger, the sirtfood diet can help you to make immense progress in the long-run by helping you to consistently shed your fat deposits while consolidating on your muscle mass gains.

3. Should I continue with the Sirtfood Diet after hitting my Target Weight?

The aim of the sirtfood diet is to help you to build a healthy routine that would allow you to stay healthy and disease-free in the long term. Even after reaching your target weight, try as much as possible to keep sirtfoods dominant in your diet, and avoid forbidden foods such as alcohol and processed sugar as much as possible. Sticking to the basic rules will help prevent you from gaining excess weight again. Remember to also keep exercising and going for regular medical check-ups if necessary.

4. **How many times should I drink the Sirtfood Green Juice per day?**

This is quite a common question among people who are just getting familiar with the sirtfood diet. Because of the intense calorie restriction in the first three days of phase one, it is recommended that you consume three cups of the sirtfood green juice per day for those three days. For the subsequent four days of Phase One, the sirtfood juice can be consumed twice per day. From phase 2 onwards, it is okay to keep the consumption of the juice at one cup per day; to be taken before breakfast in the morning to help give you your daily dose of green vitality.

5. **Can I embark on the Sirtfood Diet if I'm on special medication?**

If you are using meds, then you might need to talk to your doctor before starting the diet. However, even if your meds wouldn't allow you to go through the intense calorie restrictions of phase one, you can still incorporate sirtfoods into your diet and enjoy the amazing goodness that comes from consuming these foods.

6. **Can Pregnant women embark on the sirtfood diet?**

Once again, try as much as possible to talk to your physician before making any decisions on the sirtfood diet as a pregnant woman. Your baby requires enough nutrition as possible, and restricting calories in this delicate stage may not be such a good idea. You can, however, incorporate the sirtfoods into your diet also. Children also should not embark on a full-scale diet. Instead, they should just be fed a lot of sirtfoods.

7. **Must I complete the Seven-day period of Phase One?**

For superlative execution, it is recommended that the seven-day period for phase One be completed. However, if for health reasons or any other cogent excuse, you cannot complete the full days, then try to stick to the rules of phase One for a minimum of five days to reap the rewards of the sirtfood diet. If you have a special medical condition such as ulcers, talk to your doctor before embarking on this diet, or simply just incorporate sirtfoods into your regular diet. Note that if you want to repeat the first phase of the diet, you have to wait for a month before going through that seven-day regimen again.

CHAPTER TWELVE

SUMMARY

In this book, we have examined, in great detail, the novel and extremely effective sirtfood diet. In the opening chapter, we promised to go over the mechanism of action of the sirtfood diet, the benefits of the diet, the foods that make up the diet, a shopping list for the foods, recipes for the foods in the sirtfood diet, success stories, a meal plan, and answers to burning questions you might have. Wehave managed to go through all that and even more. The ball is in your court right now, and it is up to you to put the information that you have garnered from this book into good use. It is not too unusual for people to consume revolutionary information and not put them to good use. A lot of times, it takes just one book or one piece of information to change your life, and to be honest, this book could be your turning point.

The sirtfood diet is so effective because its effects are noticed almost immediately, spurring you on to keep trying to make more progress. As has been described extensively in the book, the foods in the diet are packed with nutrients and biochemicals called polyphenols that would work in tandem with the calorie-restriction policy to help to activate a special set of genes in your body called the sirtuins. The sirtuins would then direct a series of biochemical reactions in your body, which would help to instigate the burning of accumulated fat deposits, enhance fitness and mental alertness, and reduce your susceptibility to chronic diseases in the long term.

The foods that make up the sirtfood diet have also been shown to contain other extremely helpful biochemicals such as antioxidants that help to counteract the effects of free radicals on the body, thereby helping to slow down aging. The anticarcinogenic agents in most of the core sirtfoods help to reduce the risk of cancer. Most of the sirtfoods also contain anti-inflammatory agents that help to prevent inflammations in the long and short term. The sirtfoods are also loaded with a lot of nutrients, which help to boost the immune system, lower blood sugar, correct and manage bone defects and promote the long-term well-being of the human body.

The possibilities that the sirtfood diet offers are practically endless. This is a fortuity for you to make a difference in your life by making a difference to work on what goes into your body. You want to be fit, trim, healthy, and mentally alert? Think about how much more information you could recall and retain, how much you could save in hospital bills, and how much you could achieve with a fitter body. The choice is yours, but I would advise you to get started on this diet right away. Fortune awaits the bold ladies and gentlemen, and finally, I'd like to use this medium to welcome you to a world of uncountable opportunities. Welcome to the Sirtfood Diet!

CPSIA information can be obtained
at www.ICGtesting.com
Printed in the USA
LVHW012321100121
675857LV00005B/449

9 781801 142663